Nurse Retention Toolkit

Everyday Ways to
Recognize and Reward Nurses

Lydia Ostermeier, MSN, RN, CHCR
Bonnie Clair, BSN, RN

Nurse Retention Toolkit: Everyday Ways to Recognize and Reward Nurses is published by HCPro, Inc.

HCPro, Inc., provides information resources for the healthcare industry.

MAGNET™, MAGNET RECOGNITION PROGRAM®, and ANCC MAGNET RECOGNITION® are trademarks of the American Nurses Credentialing Center (ANCC). The products and services of HCPro, Inc. and The Greeley Company are neither sponsored nor endorsed by the ANCC.

HCPro, Inc., is not affiliated in any way with The Joint Commission, which owns the JCAHO and Joint Commission trademarks.

Bonnie Clair, BSN, RN, Contributing Author
Lydia Ostermeier, MSN, RN, CHCR, Contributing Author
Cameran Erny, Editor
Jamie Gisonde, Executive Editor
Emily Sheahan, Group Publisher
Patrick Campagnone, Cover Designer
Mike Mirabello, Senior Graphic Artist

Michael Roberto, Layout Artist
Audrey Doyle, Copy Editor
Liza Banks, Proofreader
Darren Kelly, Books Production Supervisor
Susan Darbyshire, Art Director
Jean St. Pierre, Director of Operations

Advice given is general. Readers should consult professional counsel for specific legal, ethical, or clinical questions. Arrangements can be made for quantity discounts. For more information, contact:

HCPro, Inc.
P.O. Box 1168
Marblehead, MA 01945
Telephone: 800/650-6787 or 781/639-1872
Fax: 781/639-2982
E-mail: *customerservice@hcpro.com*

Visit HCPro at its World Wide Web sites:
www.hcpro.com and *www.hcmarketplace.com*

08/2008
21512

Contents

Part 1: Free and budget-friendly rewards

Part 2: Foster a retention culture focused on nurses' needs

Part 3: Long-term strategies for retention

List of Figures

About the Contributors

Bonnie Clair, BSN, RN

Bonnie Clair, BSN, RN, is the retention project manager at CoxHealth in Springfield, MO. She has been a nurse for 27 years, and her clinical background includes staff nurse, charge nurse, preceptor, nurse manager, neonatal flight nurse, nursing educator, and nursing school administrator. Her bedside nursing experience encompasses medical-surgical, neuroscience, and neonatal intensive care.

Clair recently facilitated a group of staff RNs in researching and developing a clinical ladder to recognize and reward nursing excellence. She has also been involved with a steering committee to research and implement a shared governance model at CoxHealth. Clair is passionate about improving the bedside practice environment for nurses and patients.

Lydia Ostermeier, MSN, RN, CHCR

Lydia Ostermeier, MSN, RN, CHCR, is the director of nurse recruitment, retention, workforce development, resource allocation, and customer service at Clarian Health in Indianapolis, IN. She joined Clarian in 1987 and has been in her current role since 2002. In addition to recruiting and retaining more than 5,000 nurses,

Ostermeier manages contingent labor resources for the Clarian system, providing 350 internal resource pool nurses to Clarian's urban and suburban hospitals.

Ostermeier currently serves as the North Central Regional Chair for the National Association for Health Care Recruitment and is president of the Indiana Association for Health Care Recruitment. She was one of the first in the state of Indiana to become certified in healthcare recruitment. Additionally, Ostermeier spoke about the aging healthcare work force at the 2006 ANCC Magnet Recognition Program® Conference and published an article on reengineering nurse recruitment and retention for the American Organization of Nurse Executives.

How to use *Nurse Retention Toolkit: Everyday Ways to Recognize and Reward Nurses* CD-ROM

How to use the files on your CD-ROM

To adapt any of the files to your own facility, simply follow the instructions below to open the CD.

If you have trouble reading the forms, click on "View," and then "Normal." To adapt the forms, save them first to your own hard drive or disk (by clicking "File," then "Save as," and changing the system to your own). Then change the information to fit your facility, and add or delete any items that you wish to change.

The following file names correspond with tools listed in the book:

File name	Document
Fig 1-1	Figure 1.1: Excellence in Direct-Patient Care Award
Fig 2-1	Figure 2.1: Newspaper "Bragging" Story Template
Fig 2-2	Figure 2.2: Certificate
Fig 2-3	Figure 2.3: You Got Caught!
Fig 4-2	Figure 4.2: Mentor Application
Fig 4-3	Figure 4.3: Mentor Relationship Guide
Fig 5-2	Figure 5.2: Sample Employee Favorite List
Fig 5-3	Figure 5.3: Retention Survey

File name	Document
Fig 5-4	Figure 5.4: Nursing Satisfaction Questions
Fig 6-1	Figure 6.1: Praise a Peer!
Fig 6-2	Figure 6.3: Team Assessment
Fig 7-2	Figure 7.2: Retention Budget Planning Worksheet
Fig 8-1	Figure 8.1: Goals Worksheet

The following file name is only on the CD-ROM:

File name	Document
A-Quotes	Inspirational quotes
B-Giraffe	Sticking your neck out award

Installation instructions

This product was designed for the Windows operating system and includes Word files that will run under Windows 95/98 or greater. The CD will work on all PCs and most Macintosh systems. To run the files on the CD-ROM, take the following steps:

1. Insert the CD into your CD-ROM drive.
2. Double-click on the "My Computer" icon, next double-click on the CD drive icon.
3. Double-click on the files you wish to open.
4. Adapt the files by moving the cursor over the areas you wish to change, highlighting them, and typing in the new information using Microsoft Word.
5. To save a file to your facility's system, click on "File" and then click on "Save As." Select the location where you wish to save the file and then click on "Save."
6. To print a document, click on "File" and then click on "Print."

Introduction

Although there may not be a quick fix to the nursing shortage, as a nursing leader you can stop the revolving door and retain your top talent.

Nursing turnover can cost as much as 6% of a hospital's operating budget. Thus, organizations are feeling mounting pressure to retain their nursing staff.

But in a healthcare environment of ever-increasing difficulties ranging from more acute patients to diminishing reimbursement, where nurses report being busier and more stressed than ever before, how can organizations keep nurses happy, engaged, and most important, retained at their facility?

Research has shown that nurses who feel valued, appreciated, and respected—and who enjoy professional communication and working relationships—will stay at an organization and remain engaged in their profession. And there is evidence linking the highest nursing excellence award—American Nurses Credentialing Center Magnet Recognition Program® designation—to increased retention rates (Aiken 2002). Although a culture of nursing excellence is valuable to keeping nurses at the bedside, managers also play a key role in creating a culture where nurses want to stay, as well as building relationships where nurses feel important and vital to the team. Recognizing and rewarding nurses does not have to be complicated, time-consuming, or expensive. And it just got easier with this book, which offers quick and simple tips to show your nurses you value them. By learning straightforward ways to promote nursing excellence, create dynamic and supportive teams, and encourage professional development, you will foster an environment where nurses feel important and appreciated every day.

Whether you're looking for unique ways to say thank you or opportunities for some fun, keep this book on your desk and refer to it for practical tips and tools you can use every day. And for quick, inspiring ways to recognize nurses, flip through the "proven pearls," a selection of best practices from your peers.

> *"Human beings need to be recognized and rewarded for special efforts. You don't even have to give them much. What they want is tangible proof that you really do care about the job they're doing. The reward is really just a symbol of that."*

> –Tom Cash, senior vice president for American Express

Reference

Aiken, L.H. (2002). "Superior outcomes for magnet hospitals: The evidence base." In M.L. McClure & A.S. Hinshaw (Eds.), *Magnet Hospitals Revisited: Attraction and Retention of Professional Nurses.* Washington, DC: American Nurses Publishing.

Part 1

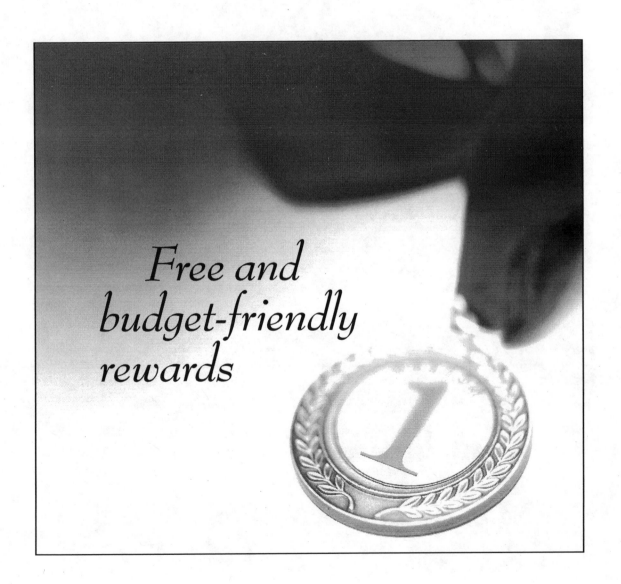

Free and budget-friendly rewards

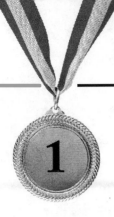

Celebrate Nurses without Breaking the Bank

On-the-Spot Recognition

Recognizing and rewarding nurses should not be a once-a-year event during Nurses Week; it should be a part of every unit's culture. But don't fret about stretching your department's meager budget. Many nurses enjoy receiving small gifts such as movie tickets, scented lotions, or gift certificates. Because whether you are showing recognition to nurses in your department or building relationships with other departments, recognition can be cost effective.

This chapter discusses low-cost strategies to help you celebrate your nurses' success, thank them for a job well done, or just let them know you're thinking about them.

Post-it power

Post-it notes are an indispensable tool for managers, allowing you to leave quick reminders for yourself or notes for others. Use the same tactic to leave a note that says something nice. Post-it notes are available in an array of designs to fit many personalities and interests. What do your employees like? Find Post-it notes that feature dogs, kittens, cooking, or sailing, or customize your own (check out Vista Print at *www.vistaprint.com*), and then leave your employees a note thanking them, telling them you noticed they did a good job, or simply letting them know you're glad they're on your team.

You can also personalize Post-it notes (check out Personalization Mall at *www.personalizationmall.com*) with a nurse's name or a simple inscription saying something like "Great work!" Write a quick note of praise to the employee on the top sheet and then place the entire stack in the employee's mailbox or on his or her desk. Every time the employee uses those notes, he or she will remember your thank you and will know that you appreciate him or her.

Proven Pearls

We are starting a banner that will be placed in the cafeteria. Anyone can write a little note on theme-shaped Post-it notes to recognize someone who did something positive on the unit or anywhere in the hospital; they can then place the note on the banner. Every quarter we plan to remove the notes and change the theme. The Post-it notes will be passed out to that employee's supervisor to be placed in a thank you card and given back to the employee.

—Carolee Hager, RNC, staff education coordinator at Pratt Regional Medical Center in Pratt, KS

Sugar magic

It's easy to make people smile if you give them treats. But don't just bring in a box of doughnuts—personalizing the treat makes it meaningful and memorable. Take a look at the following tips, some of which you can prepare in advance so you are ready whenever a member of your team goes above and beyond:

- Attach a handwritten thank you note to a basket filled with candy bars. The recipient can share the treats and the note can be posted for everyone to appreciate.

- Give a roll of Life Savers candy to a staff member who comes in to work an extra shift, and tell the staff member he or she is a "lifesaver."

- Provide a Nestlé Crunch bar to a nurse who went above and beyond his or her usual duties, along with a note saying "Thanks for helping out in a crunch!"

- Place a bunch of bananas (and other assorted fruit) in the staff break room at the start of each shift with a note saying "You are a great bunch to work with!"

- Recognize nurse involvement in interdisciplinary patient-centered organizational committees by holding a pizza party for the unit.

Proven Pearls

During Medical-Surgical Nurses Week we celebrate every day with pizza, ice cream sundaes, a home-cooked buffet, and goodie bags. I also have a $25 budget line for each nurse, so I have around a $500–$800 budget that I can do what I want with. But our nurses want a luncheon, so that's what we use the money for. During the luncheon we give away humorous awards, such as who had the most falls, and the nurse is presented with a picture of herself falling.

**—Beth Kessler, RN, director of a med-surg unit at
Lehigh Valley Hospital and Health Network in Allentown, PA**

Points mean prizes

A program that takes a little more effort to put together, but can pay huge dividends, is a recognition and reward point system. You can create a simple one among the staff on your unit, or work with the organization as a whole to create a more elaborate program that can be used across the facility. Points can be awarded for behavior such as helping out in a staffing emergency or for helping out, without being asked, a new staff member who is still getting used to your unit. Points could also be tied into professional development, such as rewards for passing certification or just for bringing in an evidence-based article the person found interesting and sharing it with colleagues.

Whatever the criteria, the points must be tied to rewards, which can be as simple or elaborate as you want. If the point system is just on your unit, consider using buttons or marbles as points, and having rewards be relevant to your unit, such as having you cover their shift for a half hour so they can take a break or a subscription to a nursing journal covering your speciality.

     Nurse Retention Toolkit

If the point system is more elaborate, consider having nurses save points to cash in for awards such as cafeteria coupons or certificates for a local spa. Consider these best practices:

- Make the point system an on-the-spot recognition program in which nurses can earn points for specific behaviors and can reward each other points for jobs well done or for helping each other out

- Consider options to earn points for performance improvement initiatives or professional development achievements, which can be cashed in for gift cards to local merchants, restaurants, or theaters

- Keep a stash of $5 gift cards on hand to reward floating nurses who may not be part of the point program

Proven Pearls

We are working on a point system where [employees] can earn points for doing good things such as working an extra shift, helping out in another unit, or floating without complaint. These bonus points can be turned in for items they can order from a book. Or, they can save up points to attend a national seminar in their specialty.

—**Carolee Hager, RNC, staff education coordinator at Pratt Regional Medical Center in Pratt, KS**

We have a system of acknowledging colleagues and coworkers for acts of kindness and helpfulness by giving a "value check," which is a 3 x 7 piece of blue paper with room to write in comments and commendations. Associates can then collect value checks and cash them in for items such as $5 restaurant cards, $5 department store cards, movie tickets, lunch bags, and so forth. When an employee receives a value check, it is noted in the employee's files.

—**Cecilia Lanuto, RN, BSN, clinical educator at Nemour's Children's Clinic in Orlando, FL**

Build Collegial Relationships

Working in a collegial environment is a key part of creating a positive workplace and improving retention, and small rewards or group activities help foster relationships.

Focus on building relationships between your unit and other departments with whom you work or interact:

- Have your team create a basket filled with goodies for another department in the hospital to show your appreciation for something they did. Have your entire staff sign a card and write their comments of appreciation. Some items you can include in the basket are microwave popcorn, pretzels, crackers, mini cans of soda, and aspirin. Benefits from this one act of kindness may include increased patience and respect among departments, along with an improved work relationship.

- Develop rapport among departments and build morale among the staff with a cookie exchange. Choose two or three departments your unit interacts with regularly and designate a day to exchange cookies.

Proven Pearls

We have placed baskets of blank praise cards, thank you cards, congratulation cards, and so forth in every unit of the hospital for peers, as well as patients, to send a note to an employee who was [seen] doing something praiseworthy.

—Carolee Hager, RNC, staff education coordinator at Pratt Regional Medical Center in Pratt, KS

To foster team spirit on your unit, purchase a large puzzle and give each nurse one piece of the puzzle during a meeting or place the puzzle piece in his or her mailbox. Explain that you need everyone's participation to symbolize the team fitting together. Have a designated place for the staff to begin working on the puzzle until it's completed. When it's completed hold an ice cream social in appreciation for everyone's contribution—provide the ice cream and have staff bring in their favorite toppings to create an ice cream buffet.

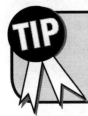 Glue the puzzle together and hang it in the unit as a reminder that the team cannot work together without everyone's input.

Build collegiality on the unit by being proud of its members. Have your staff smile for the camera and ask someone who is creative or is an amateur photographer to take candid digital photos of the staff (be careful to avoid patient faces as your staff interacts with them). Print a mix of 8 inch x 10 inch and 11 inch x 14 inch photos and purchase an assortment of frames that complement the photos. Hang the photos on a wall in your department so they are easily visible to the staff and patients. You want your patients and visitors to know that this is a great place to work, and you want potential employees to know you have a team that celebrates each other.

Proven Pearls

As an ANCC Magnet Recognition Program® (MRP) recipient in 2006, the Virginia Commonwealth University Health System in Richmond, VA, MRP champions committee wanted to educate the organization about how staff nurses exemplify the 14 Forces of Magnetism. A 10-minute video that could be shown throughout the organization was the answer.

The MRP champions found an internal videographer who understood our MRP culture and visited nursing units to film and interview staff nurses. Copies of the video are available on all nursing units for review, and they're used during nursing orientation to help newly hired nurses understand our MRP culture. The video is also given to local recruiters who are speaking with student nurses interested in coming to work for the organization.

—Rebecca Shermer, RNC, MS, clinical nurse IV, labor and delivery, and MRP champion at Virginia Commonwealth University Health System in Richmond, VA

Holiday spirit

The holidays are a time when people want to be with their families, so help them feel like their work family is important too. Sign and bake for the holidays:

- Personally sign cards during the holidays. Check outlet stores for boxed cards that are inexpensive, and allow enough time to sign each card and to write an employee name on each envelope.

- Once you are done signing the holiday cards, tie candy canes to the outside of the card with a red or green ribbon. Candy canes are available in fun and tasty flavors, such as cherry and raspberry. You can also tape Almond Joy fun-size bars to the envelope and write inside the card, "Joy to you and your family this holiday season."

- Bake or purchase loaves of bread, such as poppy seed, banana, pumpkin, or zucchini, to bring in during each shift and type the recipe on cardstock to give each nurse. This idea also works well for batches of cookies, muffins, or candy.

- Fill a holiday-themed jar with candy for a perfect gift!

Fun money

Many nurses will appreciate rewards where they can feel it most: in their wallet. Monetary recognition can take many shapes:

- Give a monetary bonus for achieving a specific percentile rank in your patient satisfaction scores.

- Give a monetary payout based on employees' individual pay scale when the organization meets its operating budget.

- Give a monetary incentive for reaching goals in the employee wellness program. (If your organization doesn't have a wellness program, have your nurses start one.)

- Give a monetary incentive for perfect attendance.

Monetary rewards don't only have to be about cold, hard cash. The payment could be in the form of a trip to an educational seminar or a bonus day or two of earned time off.

Proven Pearls

We have a perfect attendance program that gives all nursing and non-nursing staff members an opportunity to win monetary awards on a quarterly and annual basis for no missed days of scheduled work.

—Marian A. White, RN, MSN, BC, Magnet Recognition Program® project coordinator
at Memorial Hospital in Belleville, IL

Proven Pearls

We started a campaign where if you recruit a nurse, pharmacist, physical therapist, or physician you will receive $1/hour bonus pay for every hour you work, for up to two years, as long as that person remains on staff. So, if you recruited someone, you will work hard to keep him or her happy so that he or she will stay.

—Carolee Hager, RNC, staff education coordinator at Pratt Regional Medical Center in Pratt, KS

Fun and games

Establish an informal reward that can be handed out every month. For example, try a "sticking your neck out" award and give a nurse a toy giraffe for going beyond his or her usual job duties. To avoid it becoming a popularity contest, set some ground rules (e.g., no one can win more than two times per year). Be creative! A model brain could represent a "quick thinking" award; a pouch of toy gold coins can represent "you're a treasure"; and play money could represent "your actions are worth a million."

 NOTE: *Make this reward into a certificate (see the CD-ROM) with fun clipart!*

Give the stamp of approval. Create a passport from construction paper and hand out to each nurse. Nurses can get each page of the passport stamped (use a rubber stamp or stickers) by correctly answering questions regarding the unit's care-delivery model, a policy such as fall prevention, or how the unit exemplifies quality care. Once nurses receive 10 stamps, reward them with gift cards such as a free car wash.

Proven Pearls

We have a Friend of Nursing Gala that's just like the Academy Awards. Nurses are nominated and then interviewed, and winners receive monetary prizes from donors and grants. Our unit won $2,000, and we used that money to send nurses to conferences that cost less than $100; we also paid for nurses to join professional organizations. This award gave our staff an incentive to want to get more rewards.

—**Beth Kessler, RN, director on the med-surg unit at Lehigh Valley Hospital and Health Network in Allentown, PA**

RETENTION GEM: CASE STUDY

The Academy Awards for Nursing Excellence

On every ordinary day, nurses perform extraordinary service. The CNO of Grady Health System in Atlanta wanted to recognize nurses for this achievement, so Rhonda Scott, PhD, RN, created a five-star event—the Academy Awards for Nursing Excellence—to celebrate staff nurses' outstanding performance and practice.

Grady Health has been working toward creating an environment that reflects the 14 Forces of Magnetism by implementing a shared governance model, improving the image of nursing, and focusing on nurse-to-patient ratios. "We are doing all the quality expectations that go along with having an ANCC Magnet [Recognition Program® status] environment, and with this I wanted to make sure we recognized our nurses," says Scott. "We put a lot of reward and recognition activities in place with our Critical Care Nurse of the Year, Perinatal Nurse of the Quarter, and DAISY (Diseases Attacking the Immune System) Award, but our most anticipated event is our Academy Awards for Nursing Excellence."

RETENTION GEM: CASE STUDY

Nominating the champions

Grady Health is a public institution, so funds for the recognition awards were raised and donated through the hospital's foundation. In-house marketing involved save-the-date cards, flyers, posters, and brochures that were distributed throughout the hospital and to the foundation's contact list to find sponsors.

Scott created nomination forms that were distributed on every unit and anyone at Grady could nominate a staff nurse, even family members. The forms asked four questions:

1. What is the nurse's role at Grady?

2. Tell us why you think this nurse role-models nursing excellence.

3. What has this nurse done to contribute to the nursing profession (e.g., involvement in associations, national organizations, or local chapters)?

4. What else about this nurse makes him or her excellent? (For example, one nurse at Grady taught CPR to a Boy Scout group.)

Nurses could be nominated in several categories:

- LPN
- APN
- Community Service

- Education and Teaching
- Nursing Leadership
- Clinical Care

Awards were also given to nurses with outstanding contributions in ambulatory, critical care, emergency, long-term care, med-surg, oncology, perinatal, perioperative, psychiatric/mental health, and surgical areas.

RETENTION GEM: CASE STUDY

Tallying the votes

More than 200 nominations were received and distributed to 10 judges for review. The judges included a pharmacist, a nutritionist, a case management social worker, unit directors, and a businessperson from the community who was familiar with Grady nurses. Nominees' names were obscured on the forms so that the judges did not know who they were reading about, and each of the four answers from the preceding questions was individually scored. Each nominee had to be a staff nurse at Grady for two years and a full-time employee in good standing for his or her nomination to be reviewed.

Scott wanted an objective tallying of the votes, so she sent the scores to an accounting firm to be totaled. "I always want our nurses to be able to trust the integrity of this program and really believe that everyone has a chance of winning based on what they bring to the table in terms of excellence," she says. The accounting firm certified the top three finalists and the winner in each category. Out of 239 nominations, the list was narrowed to 37 finalists. Scott knew who the three finalists were for each category, so she filmed them working and took a picture for the program booklet.

Rolling out the red carpet

The 37 finalists and their guests had free admission to the awards ceremony at The Four Seasons Atlanta Hotel, whereas other attendees paid $100 for their tickets. Scott had hoped that 250 people would attend, but the event was so popular that almost 300 people attended. "A few of our physicians even wrote checks for $1,000 and told me to send 10 nurses from their unit to the awards ceremony," says Scott.

The finalists and their guests enjoyed a cocktail hour until the ballroom doors opened for the finalists to triumphantly parade in, accompanied by Tina Turner's song "Simply the Best." The event was a glittering occasion, and guests wore formal attire, which perfectly suited the red carpet that was rolled out in the ballroom and the lavish five-course

RETENTION GEM: CASE STUDY

meal. After dinner, the finalists were escorted down the red carpet by tuxedo-dressed chief nurses from each unit the finalist represented. "I told Dr. Scott that I have been a nurse at Grady since 1968, and I don't ever remember nursing being honored," says Angelle Vuchetich, RN, CANP, manager of the infectious disease program, and winner for outstanding contributions in advanced practice nursing. "Being honored as a Grady nurse is exciting!"

The event also featured a video of all 37 finalists stating why they enjoy being a nurse at Grady, as well as a slide show of the nurses in their work environment. Following a drum roll, Scott opened the sealed envelopes where the winners' names had been written in gold ink.

"When we announced the critical care winner she began to hyperventilate and couldn't get out of her chair to come on stage," says Scott. "I thought she was going to pass out!" The overall winners of each category received a personalized glass trophy, flowers, and $500, which came from the funds that were raised. The runners-up received a plaque and a bouquet of flowers. Scott had each winner make a speech and the critical care winner could hardly speak because she was emotional, says Scott. "She had the whole room in tears; the overall speeches were priceless." After the awards ceremony, everyone took to the dance floor until midnight when the ballroom doors closed.

Source: HCPro's Advisor to the ANCC Magnet Recognition Program®, *2007.*

Nurses Week Celebrations

For many nurses, Nurses Week is the highlight of their year. Many feel it is the one time of year they are confident of being appreciated and recognized for their hard work. As this book discusses, retention activities should be conducted year round and nurses should frequently hear they are appreciated and recognized. But that doesn't mean you can forget about Nurses Week! This is still a very special week, and the time of year you need to put even more thought into nurse recognition:

- Have a craft fair where nurses can bring in quilts, scrapbooking pages, jewelry, and so on for staff to purchase.

- Serve ice cream during lunch breaks.

- Invite a guest speaker to discuss professional advancement or quality care.

- Serve breakfast, lunch, or dinner for each shift.

- Distribute a bag of popcorn to every nurse.

- Have a potluck where nurses bring in their favorite dish.

- Bring a massage specialist in for a few hours and give each nurse 15 or more minutes for a massage.

- Hand out gifts such as totes, thermal lunch bags, or water bottles.

- Create T-shirts with the hospital's logo or fun nurse sayings (check out Cafe Press at *www.cafepress.com/nursing*).

- Make a DVD of your staff in action by making a slide show from digital photos. Ask the staff to e-mail you digital pictures of their peers (minus the patients) and then e-mail the photos to your IT department. Choose songs for background music and run the slide show during Nurses Week.

- Increase the visibility of nursing and nurses in your community by talking with local media.

Proven Pearls

We discovered that nurses wanted the chance to celebrate and recognize another unit in the hospital, so each unit was given a different unit to highlight during Nurses Week. They took pictures, interviewed nurses, gathered fun statistics (e.g., number of patients treated, longevity of nurses, and total years of experience), and with this they each made trifold posters. On Wednesday of Nurses Week, we displayed all of these posters in our auditorium and invited everyone to come down and look at them. The week after Nurses Week we displayed the posters in our main lobby. A lot of pride went into these posters, and it gave nurses an opportunity to go out and learn something about another unit.

—Gina Boring, MSN, RN, NE-BC, Magnet Recognition Program® director
at Aultman Health Foundation in Canton, OH

During Nurses Week, we celebrate excellence in direct patient care with an award (see Figure 1.1). Our quality of work-life council devised the award for all nurses at Fairview Ridges Hospital to recognize and award their professional behaviors and achievements. All staff nurses must be nominated by a peer and meet specific criteria, and the council reads the nominations and selects the winners (all nominees' names are blinded during the selection process). The winners are announced during Nurses Week, and they receive the opportunity to attend a national conference of their choice. And due to the high number of nominees, we have one nurse winner per cluster of units (i.e., critical care cluster, medical-surgical cluster, etc.), so we end up with eight nurses attending a national conference.

—Sue Miller, RN, MS, CNABC, director of professional practice, applied research,
and innovation at Fairview Ridges Hospital in Burnsville, MN.

| Figure 1.1 | **Excellence in Direct-Patient Care Award** |

Name of care provider: _____ **Job class:** _____

The above named person is being nominated for the Excellence in Direct-Patient Care Award for the _____ dept. of [insert hospital]. Please provide detailed examples that describe how this individual meets the criteria for each category. Comments are required for each section.

Effectively manages time

Comments: _____

_____

_____

Fosters teamwork

Comments: _____

_____

_____

Works to build a wide knowledge base

Comments: _____

_____

_____

Takes a positive "can do" attitude

Comments: _____

_____

_____

| Figure 1.1 | Excellence in Direct-Patient Care Award (cont.) |

Demonstrates problem-solving skills

Comments: _____
_____
_____

Demonstrates the importance of a diverse approach to patient care

Comments: _____
_____
_____

Provides consistent and exceptional patient and family education:

Comments: _____
_____
_____

Demonstrates critical thinking

Comments: _____
_____
_____

Demonstrates understanding of the nurse's role as a patient advocate

Comments: _____
_____
_____

Figure 1.1	**Excellence in Direct-Patient Care Award (cont.)**

Demonstrates ability to coordinate care for patients

Comments: _____

_____

_____

This employee has no performance problems or work-rule violations.

Manager's signature: _____ Date: _____

Staff member's signature: _____

Nominator's signature: _____

Source: Sue Miller, RN, MS, CNABC, director of professional practice, applied research, and innovation at Fairview Ridges Hospital in Burnsville, MN. Used with permission.

Personalize Gifts and Party Favors

During Nurses Week and beyond, when it's time to celebrate nursing excellence with gift certificates, lapel pins, or fun gifts such as a stethoscope pin, the gift will mean even more if it's personalized, and there are many helpful Web sites where you can personalize all your nursing needs. And don't forget about party celebrations for birthdays or for Nurses Week where you will need themed items and prizes.

The following Web sites offer personalized gifts, party favors, and stress relievers.

Baudville (*www.baudville.com*)

Let your nurses know they are appreciated with a variety of sizes and styles of lanyards, certificates, stickers, key chains, personalized greeting cards, tote bags, lapel pins, and much more. And don't forget to sign up for Baudville's free retention tips e-newsletter.

Positive Promotions (*www.positivepromotions.com*)

For those times when you want to give unique rewards, Positive Promotions has stethoscope lapel pins, badge holders that say "Nurses touching lives one person at a time," and buttons that say "Committed to excellence," along with gifts you can personalize.

Select-A-Gift (*www.selectagift.com*)

If you want to start a point system for perfect attendance or professional development, use Select-A-Gift's point system and give nurses the opportunity to choose their own prize. Select-A-Gift's points are valued at 50 cents each, so if a nurse earns 5,000 points, it equals $25 that he or she can redeem online.

Fun Express (*www.funexpress.com*)

Celebrating nurses' birthdays or throwing a themed party for appreciation just became more exciting with Fun Express, because you can find party decorations to go along with the theme, as well as party favors.

Trainers Warehouse (*www.trainerswarehouse.com*)

Trainers Warehouse will help you ease new-nurse jitters with ice breaker games, or give nurses a way to relieve stress with unique stress toys in a variety of shapes, including a star, hot potato, and light bulb.

Branders (*www.branders.com*)

Everything you want to personalize for nurses is just a click away, from pens, stress balls, and hats to apparel, Post-it notes, mouse pads, and much more.

Identity Links (*www.identity-links.com*)

If you want a site that specializes in promotional nurse-specific rewards, Identity Links is your go-to place, offering ambulance stress relievers, nurse memo holders, heart-shaped pedometers, and many more nurse-specific ideas. Your nurses will be sure to thank you.

Motivators (*www.motivators.com/Promotional-NursesWeek-Products-61.html*)

Prepare for Nurses Week with these nursing promotional items. Whether you choose the chocolates, nurse business card sculpture, or relaxation aromatherapy kit, this site is a great way to celebrate nurses.

RETENTION GEM: BUDGET-FRIENDLY GIFTS

Twenty budget-friendly gifts for any occasion:

- Pocket or wall calendar

- $5 gift certificate to the hospital gift shop

- Coupon for a free ice cream in the cafeteria

- Potted plant

- Ball cap for a local sports team

- Coffee mug

- Logo pens

- Candle

- Magnets for the refrigerator

- Nurse-themed book or bookmark

- Keychain

- Scented soap, lotion, or bubble bath

- Stationery

- Homemade cookies

- Microwave popcorn

- Disposable camera with a photo album

- Gourmet nuts

- Journal

- Address book

- Gas card

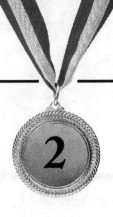

No-Cost, Everyday Ways to Recognize and Reward Nurses

2

LEARNING OBJECTIVES

After reading this chapter, the participant will be able to:

- Identify simple and free ways to reward staff

- Identify local resources to recognize staff

- Recognize ways to have fun while working

Crafting a Caring Environment

Creating an environment where nurses feel appreciated, valued, and that they are making a positive impact on patient care is a key to improving retention. Just as important is building a trusting and respectful relationship between managers and staff.

How do you make nurses feel vital to the organization or the department they are in? How do you help them feel significant in their role? There are many simple things managers can do to turn around staff members' perceptions and help them feel they are vital to the organization. And none of them have to cost any money—all that matters are that the communication and recognition is sincere and that the message or reward means something to the nurse being recognized.

Everyday rewards

Strategies you can use every day include the following:

- Ask your director or vice president of nursing to stop by and compliment one or more of your staff members on something they have accomplished. This lets nurses know you have been speaking positively about them to your boss, who is someone they probably don't see very often.

- Invite a staff person into your office just to say "thank you" for a specific behavior or excellent intervention he or she provided for a patient or family. Let the staff member know you noticed, and refrain from discussing any other departmental issues.

- Get a flip chart that has a sticky strip on the back so you can hang it on the wall. Every week or so, write a sentence or two of recognition for something an employee did: "Thanks Sally, you handled that difficult family last week with skill and compassion"; "Great job getting that equipment repaired in a timely manner, Mike. I know the staff appreciated your hard work"; "Nancy, you really helped our staffing crunch by coming in for extra hours last Friday."

- Hang a flip chart in the staff lounge area and ask staff to recognize a peer. Before it's time to flip the chart to start over, allow the recognized employee to keep the compliments he or she received from peers.

- Walk by your employees' work space or their lockers; do they have personal photos posted? Are awards or certificates posted, and do you know the details surrounding them? Taking note of these things and commenting on them connects you to your staff and helps staff members feel like an important part of the group.

 Nurse Retention Toolkit

- Create a surprise hour off once per week, month, or quarter, and choose an employee whose assignments you will take over for that hour. Say "I appreciate the way you handled . . . and I would like to reward you by giving you an hour for lunch/dinner. Take an hour today and come back refreshed!"

Proven Pearls

As a unit-level manager, I, along with the other clinical partner, recognize little things often. That is to say that we laud accomplishments, share sorrows, care for those who are ill, and mark milestones. We all sign cards and often write personal notes. If your birthday, employment anniversary, child's graduation, and Nurses Week all fall in the same month, you will get four cards and maybe some flowers! We make our staff feel cared for like family.

—**Ginger Brooks, RN, BSN, OR clinical partner in Labor and Delivery at Greater Baltimore Medical Center in Baltimore**

Make the Most of Staff Meetings

Unit staff meetings are usually full of agenda points regarding vital information that our nurses must know. As such, it's easy to forget the importance of recognizing staff nurses during a time when all their peers are in one room to hear and congratulate. Don't put nurse recognition on the back burner at staff meetings—take this valuable opportunity to celebrate nurses' excellence:

- Draw one staff name out of a hat during each unit meeting, and designate that person as Employee of the Month for that month. This allows everyone equal opportunity and avoids being a popularity contest. Give the rest of the staff a predetermined amount of time to e-mail or write down their "kudos" about that nurse. Either you or someone on staff (a creative person who loves crafts, art, design, etc.) can put the comments together to be presented to the recognized employee at the next staff meeting—before you draw the next person's name. Comments can be compiled and typed on a certificate or even on a scrapbook page to create a collage. And remember the following:

- Staff members can get their name in the hat only if they attend the meeting

- Post the monthly comments from peers in plain view on your unit to offer great peer recognition

- No one can "win" more than once unless every staff member has had the opportunity to be Employee of the Month

- Put out a bulleted memo containing all the information you need to go over in your monthly unit staff meetings, and then you can devote your scheduled meeting time to a particular topic, such as "What's on your mind?" Don't create an agenda—just make time for you and your staff to connect. Tell staff members to bring their favorite soft drink or coffee.

- Increase participation and ownership in staff meetings by posting a blank agenda in the nurses' lounge a week before the scheduled meeting. Staff members can post questions, concerns, or desired discussions. You may even become aware of issues you previously didn't know about.

- Begin each staff meeting with recognition of staff members mentioned on patient satisfaction surveys or in thank you cards from patients.

- Hand out staff awards at each staff meeting. Throughout the month, have staff members e-mail you about something great a coworker has done. At the end of the staff meeting, recognize those staff members.

Publicize Your Nurses

Is there an area in your department that you can reserve for noting accomplishments? An easy way to recognize the nursing staff and show your appreciation is to use local resources: bulletin boards, newspaper ads, and the Web sites for your organization as a whole, as well as the dedicated nursing Web site.

Use a dry erase board in your break room to jot notes of "thanks" or "job well done." And encourage staff members to write notes to each other and to designate one nurse to clear the board each week so it stays current. Here are some additional suggestions:

- Provide a link to the nursing Web site from the hospital home page

- Select a nurse to highlight on the nursing Web site every month

- Find an old shelving unit that's not being used a create a display case that features awards won by staff nurses

- Develop and display an Employee of the Month bulletin board

- When you're placing a recruitment ad in the local newspaper, include a picture of a seasoned nurse with a comment recognizing the nurse for all that he or she has done at the organization

Proven Pearls

Nurses who achieve employee of the month or year are recognized throughout the year with their picture and a feature article in a community publication. We also feature nurses in cable ads and advertisements for health fairs.

—**Marian A. White, RN, MSN, BC, Magnet Recognition Program®
project coordinator at Memorial Hospital in Belleville, IL**

Take advantage of local resources

Brag about your nurses every chance you get. As organizations, we do not brag enough about all the accomplishments that our nursing staff is able to complete, whether it's meeting patient safety goals or recognizing OR nurses who just received their OR certification. See Figure 2.1 and get some bragging going on in your local community newspapers.

Figure 2.1	Newspaper "Bragging" Story Template

ABC hospital is pleased to announce two surgical nurses recently completed their specialty certifications. After providing a preliminary course to prepare for the intensive written exam, ABC hospital sponsored the nurses who both successfully passed the challenge.

Their completion demonstrates a commitment to patient excellence, as well as a desire to maintain a higher knowledge level of their specialty. ABC hospital is proud of our nursing staff and supports their efforts in developing their professionalism and education.

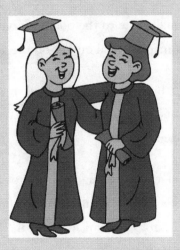

Tip:

• Include a photo of the nurses holding their certificates

• Print their individual names under the image

• Include manager in photo congratulating them

Source: Shelley Cohen, RN, BS, CEN, founder and president of Health Resources Unlimited, www.hru.net, in Tennessee. Reprinted with permission.

Hang bulletin boards

Hang bulletin boards in your department that feature unique information and have themes that are fun for everyone to see. Nurses today receive so many mandatory flyers and memos—even the restroom has become a place for reading. Here are a few ideas for creating a themed bulletin board:

- Make it seasonal. Find a staff RN who has an interest in creative design. Have him or her be in charge of changing the scenery on your board every month.

- Add an inspirational quote to the board every week (take a look at 30 great examples of inspirational quotes on the accompanying CD-ROM).

- Highlight staff birthdays, tenure with your organization, or an exciting vacation. If someone gets married or has a baby/grandchild, highlight those important events as well.

- Post a "Guess who" contest using baby photos or nursing school graduation photos. You could have small prizes for the most correct guesses. You could even open it up to patients and visitors if the board is on the unit rather than in the staff lounge.

- Post a "Guess the pet owner" contest. This allows staff members a small glimpse into the outside lives of peers, which helps them to feel like they are connected to coworkers.

- Use wrapping paper on the board for a variety of background themes.

- Staple items to the board to add dimension, such as silk flowers, plastic ivy, scrapbook embellishments, or anything from a craft store.

 Nurse Retention Toolkit

- Feature nursing-related problem-solving questions each month on a bulletin board. Write out a problem at the top of the board and have colorful Post-it notes available for staff to write their solution along with their name and stick it on the board. To avoid having to analyze solutions yourself, ask your unit-based practice council to select the best solution and then announce it during a staff meeting. Have the winner who best answered the nursing problem-solving question discuss his or her solution during the staff meeting as a best practice for their peers to use.

- Provide a sense of camaraderie for staff members by allowing them to collaborate on creating themes for the bulletin board. Here are few ideas that your staff, patients, and visitors will enjoy:

  – "Cruise into our unit" or "Cruise into your best health." Include pertinent health information for your patient population and decorate the board with boats or sailboats, a pier, a dock, anchors, lifesavers, and water.

  – "Instruments of health." Decorate with music notes, sheet music, toy musical instruments, Symphony candy bar wrappers, and music scales.

  – "It's time for your best health." Decorate with pictures of clocks, calendars, an hourglass, a date book, a kitchen timer, and various types of watches.

  – "Recipe for good health." Decorate with recipe cards, measuring spoons or cups, ingredients, cookie cutters, the label from a bottle of canola or olive oil, and heart-healthy cookbook covers.

– "Tools for your health" or "Nursing tools of the trade." Decorate with pictures of garden, power, lawn, or mechanical tools.

– "Sowing seeds for your good health." Decorate with packets of seeds. You might try to attach a small bag of dirt, a small watering can, or a picture of sunshine and garden tools.

Proven Pearls

We maintain a bulletin board that is just for fun. Sometimes we just have it full of funny pictures of each other (and of our doctors, as well!) and sometimes we have a theme (e.g., all staff members bring in baby pictures, or pictures from their teen years, or pictures of pets). It really makes us all feel like a family, and the patients love it too!

—**Debbie Smith, RNC, charge nurse, nursery/NICU at The Medical Center at Bowling Green in Bowling Green, KY**

We have a "brag board" where everyone is encouraged to post pictures of children, grandchildren, or pets. And to engage staff members we have contests. Our "Do you know these babies?" contest was popular. Staff members brought in baby pictures of themselves and the pictures were posted with no names attached. We submitted our guesses and the person with the most correct answers won. Many of us also have debriefing dinners or breakfasts, and we meet after work to just relax—it is camaraderie.

—**Ginger Brooks, RN, BSN, OR clinical partner in labor and delivery at Greater Baltimore Medical Center in Baltimore**

The Simple Act of a "Thank You"

Sending a thank you card or telling a nurse "thank you" for a job well done goes a long way. It's easy to get caught up in the midst of a busy day, but taking a few minutes to send a simple thank you will always be remembered.

Craft a thank you note

Before you send a personalized thank you note, follow these special guidelines:

- Use blue or black ink to offer a more professional appearance

- Begin with the recipient's name (this lets the recipient know it's a personal note, not just a form letter)

- Say "thank you"

- Be specific about the behavior or action you're recognizing:

    - "The extra hours you stayed over to help . . ."

    - "Your positive attitude in a stressful situation . . ."

    - "Your willingness to change your schedule . . ."

    - "Your going the extra mile with [patient], [family], [coworker] . . ."

- Be sure to mention the positive effect of the recipient's behavior or action:

    - "Your work/dedication made this project a huge success"

- "Your creative thinking saved our department time/resources"

- "Your faithfulness to follow through is a great example"

• Connect the recipient's behavior to your organizational mission:

- "Thanks to you, we're sure to reach our goals!"

- "Thanks to your efforts, we're on our way to achieving . . ."

• Say "thank you" again

• Close your note with a meaningful sign-off:

- "Keep up the great work, because it's being noticed!"

- "Cheers!"

- "Best regards."

• Sign your name

• To add a special flair, consider including a small treat:

- Roll of Life Savers candy (You're a lifesaver!)

- 100 Grand candy bar (Your efforts are priceless!)

- 3 Musketeers candy bar (Three cheers for you and your work!)

- Shoestring licorice (Great job in tying together that project!)

– PayDay candy bar (Your efforts will lead to a great return for our patients/department/organization!)

– M&M's (Thanks for not melting under pressure!)

Find the right words

Sometimes managers really want to start writing cards to their staff, but when they pick up a pen their mind goes blank. Here are a few ideas for you to use as a baseline, and you can craft the sentiment to go along with any of them:

- Your dedication contributes to our department's success.

- Your ability to recognize and react to opportunity has resulted in personal and departmental success.

- The service/care/concern you provided exceeded all expectations.

- Your personal commitment to excellence has inspired others.

- Thanks for coming up to bat at the end of the ninth inning.

- You took the time to make a difference.

- You consistently go the extra mile.

- What a brilliant idea! Thanks for sharing it with our department and me.

- You shine bright!

- You have a wonderful ability to really listen.

Call and write home

Even though you may have verbally said "thank you" to employees at work for something they have done above and beyond the call of duty, take the time to call them at home after their shift to thank them again. It's preferable that you make the call from your home instead of your office. You may be surprised how far this small gesture can go.

Proven Pearls

One of the things I started is sending out handwritten thank you cards to my staff at their home address. I thank them for getting caught doing something wonderful, earning an "exceeds standards" in any area of the annual evaluation, and acknowledging them as being named in a satisfaction survey for doing a great job. Staff members bring their cards in to show other staff members that they received one, and they show them to their family members. They really are proud of being noticed. I think I get more "thank you" feedback from them as they come and thank me for thanking them! Our staff retention increased from 63% in 2006 to 72.5% in 2007. I can't credit the thank you cards for all the progress, but I do have to say that I think a lot of it was from the cards.

—David Hribar, resident services director at Providence Extended Care Center in Anchorage, AK

We call discharged patients back within 72 hours, and if the patient provides a positive comment about a nurse, our administrator and I send the nurse a personal thank you note.

**—Beth Kessler, RN, director on the med-surg unit at
Lehigh Valley Hospital and Health Network in Allentown, PA**

Honor Excellence with Awards

Giving awards is a great way to encourage nurses to provide quality patient care, strive for excellence, and enhance professional skills. Awards don't have to be fancy, etched-glass trophies. The important thing is recognizing the behavior, skill, or compassion and letting the person know it's appreciated. A simple way to do this is by creating a certificate, which is easy to do with any desktop publishing software and can be customized with just the right wording. Take a look at the example in Figure 2.2. The template is included on this book's accompanying CD-ROM, so you can customize the award for any nurse in any situation.

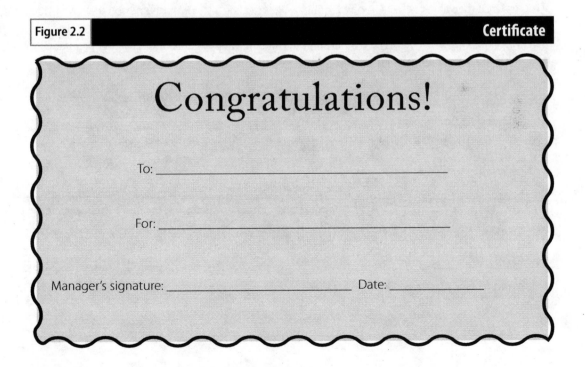

Figure 2.2	Certificate

Congratulations!

To: _____

For: _____

Manager's signature: _____ Date: _____

Try some of these best practices from your peers regarding awards presented at their organizations.

Proven Pearls

We present one staff nurse every month with the DAISY (Diseases Attacking the Immune System)—an award given by the DAISY Foundation, a nonprofit organization that recognizes the excellent patient care nurses provide every day. Staff members at Grady Health nominate a nurse by telling a specific story about the compassionate and caring side of the nurse. At the end of each month, stories regarding the nominees are brought before the nurse executive council to vote on a winner. The nominees' names are obscured so that the nurse executive council members do not know the nurses' names or the unit they work on.

The nurse executive council discloses the winner's name and unit to me and then I send out an e-mail to the entire Grady Health staff to ask them to come with the nurse executive to surprise the DAISY winner. We have this big banner that says "Congratulate our DAISY Award Winner for Compassionate and Caring Nurses," carry pompoms, and play the song "Simply the Best" by Tina Turner. Once the winner is notified on his or her unit, I read the letter from the person that nominated him or her, attach a daisy pen to his or her uniform, and then give the winner a pot of daisies to plant in his or her yard. The banner stays outside the winner's unit with his or her picture on it until the next month, when a new DAISY winner is awarded.

—**Rhonda Scott, PhD, RN, CNO at Grady Health System in Atlanta**

We have a nursing excellence award where nurses must be nominated by their peers. Nine to 12 recipients are recognized and their picture is posted prominently in our hospital newsletters.

—**Marian A. White, RN, MSN, BC, Magnet Recognition Program®**
project coordinator at Memorial Hospital in Belleville, IL

Proven Pearls

We have a monthly drawing called "You got caught!!" that features the characters from the movie *Finding Nemo*. Each month at our unit meetings we pick something we want to improve on, like charting the contact phone number or catching someone giving good customer service. When we "catch" someone doing the right thing we give him or her a certificate (see Figure 2.2), and put the person's name on one of the "Nemo" characters and place these characters in a fish bowl. At our unit meeting we have a drawing, and our manager purchases different gifts for the lucky winner of the drawing.

—**Sharon Pollok, RN, charge nurse, newborn and special care nursery at Saint John Medical Center in Tulsa, OK**

Figure 2.3	You Got Caught!

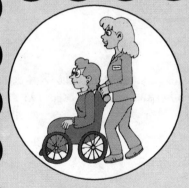

YOU have been CAUGHT!

Doing: _____

_____

Thank You!

Name: _____

Source: Sharon Pollok, RN, charge nurse in newborn and special care nursery at Saint John Medical Center in Tulsa, OK. Adapted with permission.

The Power of Relaxation and Fun Activities

In the same way that not every retention strategy has to cost money, neither does it have to take a lot of time or be serious professionalism. Lots of simple retention tips make nurses happy and entitle them to have fun.

Play ball

Do you have a local baseball team? If so, ask the team's manager whether a staff nurse from your unit can throw out the first pitch at a game. Select the lucky winner by placing staff names in a baseball hat and drawing a name.

Proven Pearls

We have a nursing volleyball team, and every year we plan a camping trip together.

—Beth Kessler, RN, director on the med-surg unit at Lehigh Valley Hospital and Health Network in Allentown, PA

Cozy up and de-stress

Do you have a small space where you can create a relaxing nook for the staff? It may be just a corner of your lunchroom or one end of your locker room. Designate that space as the relaxation nook (or make up a clever name for your unit/department, such as "No crisis zone" or "Radiology rejuvenation area"). No phone calls are allowed in the relaxation nook. Ask staff members whether anyone can donate an old couch or recliner, and have the staff bring in old magazines, a lamp, pillows, a tabletop water fountain, a clock so no one goes over his or her allotted break time, and maybe a CD player. Be creative!

Proven Pearls

One Thursday per month, the med-surg nurses meet with pastoral care for one hour, and I bring lunch for the nurses and cover the unit. This is for them to decompress and relax. It's a very powerful and quiet time.

> —**Beth Kessler, RN, director on the med-surg unit at Lehigh Valley Hospital and Health Network in Allentown, PA**

Laugh

It was a wise person who first said laughter is the best medicine:

- Station top-level management outside with buckets of soap, sponges, and hoses to wash employees' cars before they go home. It's a great way get nurses to smile and even laugh.

- Create a theme on a monthly basis for staff meetings where nurses have to dress up. The themes could be favorite action hero or movie character, sports team, or funniest wig.

- Have a Halloween costume contest where staff nurses' dress up and the winner receives a pumpkin full of candy, pumpkin bread, or a pumpkin scented candle.

- Laugh and let staff hear you chuckle! Laughter is contagious, so good moods affect others in a positive way and bad moods infect others negatively.

Proven Pearls

We are working on a book for humorous or inspiring stories written by our nurses with things that have happened to us over the years. Our plan is to go to [an online photo Web site] to make a coffee-table book.

> —**Carolee Hager, RNC, staff education coordinator at Pratt Regional Medical Center in Pratt, KS**

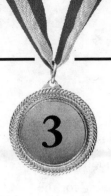

Reward and Recognition Tips to Appeal to All Generations

One Retention Tip Does Not Fit All

Savvy managers recognize that one size does not fit all for retention tips. Everyone has different preferences and motivators, and the same applies for retention techniques. It's also important to consider that the nursing work force today is the most diverse work force it has ever been and you likely have nurses from four different generations working at your organization.

Different generations tend to share some similarities and characteristics that, when understood, will help you tailor retention activities so you use ones most suitable to your employees.

The needs of four generations

1. The silents

Also called the "Greatest Generation" or the "traditionalists," the silents were born between 1926 and 1946. This generation's characteristics encompass traditional American values, and they value respect, obedience, hard work, and saving for the future. The Depression and World War II shaped the generation's formative years, instilling attributes of patriotism, loyalty, and dedication.

Five characteristics of the silent generation:

1. Good listeners and facilitators

2. Derive pleasure from a job well done

3. Loyal to the company

4. Strong work ethic

5. Adaptive

The silent generation has built up years of wisdom and expertise. So when looking at retention tips for silents, consider offering:

• Flexible schedules (read more in Chapter 5)

• Time off for holidays

• Classes to help them prepare for retirement

• Easy access to commonly needed supplies

• Centralized work stations

- Patient-lifting devices

- Training on how to use new technology

- Continual recognition and celebration for their valuable contributions

- Praise for their knowledge and expertise

2. The baby boomers

The baby boomers were born between 1946 and approximately 1962 and are currently the largest generation in the nursing work force. But in the next few years Generation Y will surpass them.

Baby boomers are influenced by the time they grew up, when the country was affluent, and are often motivated by increases in paycheck and status. Thus, they are willing to put in long hours at work. They are also affected by the social upheaval of the 1960s, leading many in the generation to question traditional authority structures. So if you want to grasp a better understanding of baby boomers, take them out for a cup of coffee to discuss the '60s and '70s.

Five characteristics of baby boomers:

1. Big risk takers and thinkers

2. Good decision-makers

3. Good mentors

4. Career minded

5. Good work ethic

Baby boomers want recognition and respect for their significant contributions. Thus, when looking at retention tips for baby boomers, consider offering:

- Flexibility for time off during the holidays

- Time away from patients to work on unit posters, unit newsletters, or quality projects

- Opportunities to work in teams

- Transitional training or educational programs to pursue further education (e.g., master's degree)

- Opportunity to become a mentor or a research assistant

- The combination of vacation and sick time into paid time off to allow boomers to use their time however they see fit

- The opportunity to plan social events

- Time-saving programs such as an onsite bank or post office

3. Generation X

Born between 1962 and 1979, this generation is sometimes called the baby busters. They are a smaller generation than the baby boomers or the generation that follows them.

Generation Xers are exceedingly independent, but can be skeptical and wary of authority. This is a generation that grew up seeing their parents lose jobs to downsizing and economic uncertainty, so their loyalty is first to themselves and their professional development, rather than to the employer for whom they work. And since this generation grew up in a changing world, they are accepting of change, difference, and diversity.

Five characteristics of generation Xers:

1. Flexible

2. Focused, goal-oriented

3. Self-reliant

4. Committed to work-life balance

5. Have their own way of doing things

Generation X believes in a fun workplace and will not often sacrifice their time and freedom for money. They want to be challenged, heard, and rewarded, so when looking at retention tips for Generation Xers, consider offering:

• Frequent training and opportunities to learn new skills

• Classes that give them skills in coping and stress management

• Mentoring relationships with older generations

• The opportunity to develop goals for the unit and the organization

• Team-building opportunities during meetings and outside of work

• Opportunities to attend a seminars for free, as well as a free day to go to them

- Frequent recognition programs (e.g., rewarding a staff nurse for excellence monthly with a monetary reward)

- Flexibility with time off to enjoy life

- Appreciation for their hard work and dedication

- Encouragement for them to share their ideas and comments

4. Generation Y

Born after 1980, the Y'ers are fast becoming the predominant generation in the work force. They are bursting on the scene now with a desire to change everything, much like the boomers of 30 years ago, and they are committed to striving for excellence and delivering strong results. They are often realistic and, like silents, tend to be very loyal. But they sometimes intimidate older workers with their openness and ability to state what's on their minds. If they do not see the value of a rule or practice, they are likely to speak up and want to change it.

Five characteristics of generation Y'ers:

1. Family-centered

2. Affectionate

3. Inspirational thinking

4. Welcome guidance

5. Volunteer readily

When looking at retention tips for this technologically-savvy generation, consider offering:

- Challenges to feed their need to work hard and deliver strong results

- Opportunity to "test drive" new technology and then coach peers on how to use it

- Internships and formalized clinical mentoring activities with coaches

- Personal fulfillment through attention on the job, feedback, and opportunities to lead

- Your personal time to answer their questions and hear their ideas

- Ongoing coaching to enhance job performance

- Flexible work options to have a work-life balance

- Support as they try new opportunities and learn new tasks

- Acceptance, even if it's just a hug

- Guidance to help them see what they want to do professionally and what they can do

Nurse's Most Valued Work-Related Recognition

With nurses representing such multigenerational diversity, managers already know that not every nurse feels the same way about all nursing issues; and in the same vein, not every nurse wants to be recognized or rewarded in the same way. It is your job to pay attention to your nurses' needs and to tailor your efforts to what they want and what resonates with them.

The following is a list of nurses of various ages, who share how they like to be recognized.

Name: Kay Timbreza, RN, CNNP
Age: 56 years old; nursing for 21 years in neonatology
Most valued work-related recognition: "When someone says 'well done' or someone is grateful that I've shown up in an emergency and the patient does well."

Name: Cole Werner, RN, BSN
Age: 51 years old; nursing for 20 years
Most valued work-related recognition: "Making a connection with a patient/ family and knowing I made a difference in their lives. Individual comments from my coworkers are also very meaningful because we tend to forget each other in all our busyness."

Name: Susan Schiman, RN
Age: 48 years old; nursing for 27 years
Most valued work-related recognition: "Notes and cards given to me by patients, peers, and my nurse manager."

Name: Phyllis Krebs, RN, BSN, CNOR

Age: 52 years old; nursing for 32 years

Most valued work-related recognition: "Being recognized as a resource for my area of nursing."

Name: Pat Clutter, RN, M.Ed, CEN, FAEN

Age: 57 years old; nursing for 36 years

Most valued work-related recognition: "Being recognized for my value as a nurse and having my boss recognize and truly utilize my talents. I value most those colleagues that I work with who treat me as they would like to be treated. Pay increases are valued as well, but not as much as these other forms of recognition."

Name: Annie Durrington, RN, BSN

Age: 25 years old; nursing for two years

Most valued work-related recognition: "When someone from upper management recognizes me for a job well done it really means a lot. I'm fairly new to management, and to know that I'm doing the job well and receiving gratitude from someone above me makes it worthwhile!"

Name: Debbie Denson, RN, BSN

Age: 48 years old; nursing for 23 years

Most valued work-related recognition: "Happy staff [members who] say 'thank you' and 'I'm glad you are here,' and administration telling me that what I am doing is valuable to them."

Name: Debra James, RN, BSN

Age: 45 years old; nursing for 24 years

Most valued work-related recognition: "A note from staff nurses or managers that my assistance in their workplace was helpful and appreciated."

Name: D'Ann Kohls, RN, BSN, M.Ed

Age: 46 years old; nursing for 26 years

Most valued work-related recognition: "The respect of my coworkers and physician, as evidenced by their display of trust, and receiving increased responsibility."

Name: Julie Zuniga, RN, BSN

Age: 48 years old; nursing for 28 years

Most valued work-related recognition: "I most value someone telling me 'thank you' for my help. Then, I value compensation. Society tends to rate value by compensation. I have worked many years, have a wealth of knowledge, have paid to further my education, and expect to be compensated as a professional."

Name: Laura Nordgren, RN, BSN

Age: 43 years old; nursing for 22 years

Most valued work-related recognition: "During our monthly unit meetings our manager has a segment to recognize staff [members] who have gone above and beyond that month. Our fellow coworkers usually applaud, but sometimes we give a standing ovation!"

Name: Jennifer Burk, RN, CEN

Age: 35 years old; nursing for four years

Most valued work-related recognition: "I need a kind word or pat on the back occasionally to feel like I am making a difference. We started handing out 'You make a difference' cards a couple [of] months ago, and I look forward to those as does the rest of the staff. It's nice to have a prize as recognition too! Having [a] great staff and great leadership makes all the difference."

Name: Latoya Compton, RN, BSN

Age: 29 years old; LPN for seven years and RN for seven months

Most valued work-related recognition: "The recognition that I value most doesn't come from awards by upper management (although those are nice), or from raises (which are also nice), but from a thank you and hugs from patients and their families who sincerely mean it."

Name: Paula Warner, RN, BSN

Age: 57 years old; LPN for 17 years and RN for six years

Current position: Staff RN, geriatric psychiatric unit; CNA instructor

Most valued work-related recognition: "Praise from my coworkers. Just having them tell me they miss me when I am on vacation makes me want to keep working with these people forever."

Name: Benjamin Kirakofe, RN, OCN

Age: 40 years old; nursing for seven years

Most valued work-related recognition: "The recognition I receive from the patients and their families."

Name: Wilma (Billie) Nelson, RN, CCRN, M.Ed

Age: 64 years old; nursing for 30 years

Most valued work-related recognition: "Acknowledgment of those times that really show how I made a difference. Genuine thanks from families and colleagues and when I am sought out for my professional input."

Name: Vickey Elkins, RN, BSN

Age: LPN for 12 years; RN for 17 years

Most valued work-related recognition: "When the patient tells me 'thank you.'"

Name: Lisa Hallam, RN, BSN, SANE

Age: 40 years old; nursing for 19 years

Most valued work-related recognition: "I value recognition from my patients the most—just a simple 'thank you' for being my nurse today and a hug go a long way. I have also saved every handwritten thank you note sent to me by hospital administration. In a hospital this size, it is remarkable to receive such a gift versus an e-mail."

Name: Debra S. Mergen, RN

Age: 44 years old; nursing for 13 years

Most valued work-related recognition: "Money! Hard work and dedication should be acknowledged with a nice paycheck. I also value a simple 'thank you' and a smile from my nurse manager. Honestly, the money is no good if you don't feel appreciated."

Name: Beverly Loven, RN, BSN, BC

Age: 53 years old; nursing for 31 years

Most valued work-related recognition: "A written note of thanks from a supervisor, recognition among peers, and a 'thank you' note from a patient and/or family."

Name: Mary Ann Kenney, RN

Age: 52 years old; LPN for seven years and RN for 25 years

Most valued work-related recognition: "I highly value recognition from my boss when she takes note of my efforts. I also value the teamwork of everyone I work with."

Name: Tracy Taylor, RN

Age: 45 years old; nursing for 25 years

Most valued work-related recognition: "Comments from staff [members] that I have been a positive influence and that I have made our new employees feel welcome."

Part 2

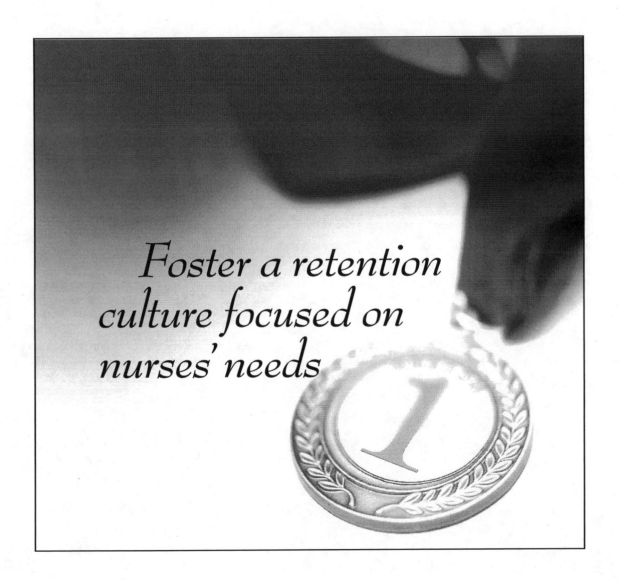

Foster a retention culture focused on nurses' needs

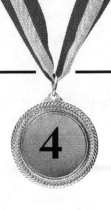

Keep New Nurse Graduates at the Bedside

Show Appreciation from the Start

Leaving nursing school to enter the work force can be a difficult transitional period for many new nurse graduates. And literature reveals that 57% of new nurse graduates will leave their first position within two years of hire (Newhouse, Hoffman, Suflita, and Hairston 2007). So, why are they leaving? Like many of us, new nurses want to feel valued, be rewarded, have a strong relationship with their manager, and enjoy a work-life balance.

Managers and their organizations expend untold time and energy recruiting and hiring new nurses, and it can be disheartening when those nurses leave so quickly. You work so hard to get nurses in the door that it makes sense to work hard to retain them. This chapter discusses strategies for helping new nurses feel welcome, comfortable, and confident of a successful future at your organization.

Welcome aboard!

Healthcare organizations know the first year of employment for a new nurse is the trickiest, so it's important to let new nurse graduates know they are welcome on the unit and will be a valued part of the team. There are a number of ways you can welcome new nurses:

- **Make welcome flyers.** Post welcome flyers around your facility—not only in nursing areas, but also in places physicians will see them.

- **Get to know them.** It can be useful to get to know new graduates before assigning them a preceptor or a mentor, because that way you have a better idea of their personality and can make a suitable placement. To accomplish this, consider spending the first two weeks of new nurses' orientation with them as much as possible.

- **Check in weekly.** Most new nurse graduates are beginning their first-ever full-time job. The reality of this can be overwhelming, so check in weekly to make sure they are not overwhelmed.

- **Go out to lunch.** Whether it's the new nurse's first or second week on the job, take the nurse out to lunch to get to know him or her. This shows nurses that you care about them.

- **Recognize the new nurse at staff meetings.** Before you begin the weekly staff meeting, take the time to introduce everyone to the new nurse. This is a great way for the new nurse to remember faces and feel a part of the team.

- **Conduct meetings.** Meet with new nurses in their first, third, and sixth months of employment to see how things are going and to establish goals and objectives for their career advancement.

A bag full of goodies

Another great way to make nurses feel welcome and valued from the get-go is to make a small welcome bag for your new hires. Their first day is sure to be stressful, so in the welcome bag include:

1. A small card to say "We are glad you are here"

2. Your business card with contact information

3. A voucher for a free cafeteria lunch

4. An organizational logo pen

5. A lapel badge holder

6. A pack of gum or candy

7. A mini bottle of hand sanitizer

And don't forget to add other interesting items and anything that pertains to your unit. For example, a neonatal flight team gives out helicopter magnets to new hires! Some fun ideas are:

1. Stress balls related to your unit (e.g., a stress ball shaped like a heart or a brain)

2. A bookmark with the organization's nursing Web site listed (See Figure 4.1)

Chapter 4

3. A small notepad for jotting down things to remember

4. Sticky notes that have a nurse-related heading such as "Nurses are patient people"

5. An organizational logo lunch bag

6. A calculator

7. A magnet illustrating the department

Figure 4.1	Nursing Web Site Bookmark

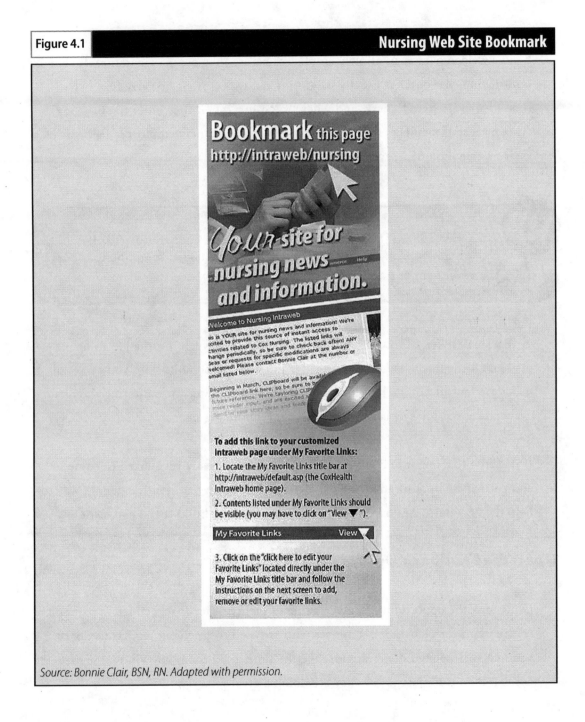

Source: Bonnie Clair, BSN, RN. Adapted with permission.

Start connections

Send a welcome letter to all new employees before they begin orientation. Include information that outlines exactly what they can expect their first day (e.g., what time to arrive, where to park, and where to go first when they enter the building). Also, have staff members sign a welcome note to make new employees feel part of their new environment, even on their first orientation day.

 Hold a social occasion in which new nurses have an opportunity to talk with their peers and get to know them. Make it a group outing to a local restaurant or a bowling alley.

Give a small token of recognition during the first few weeks on the job to help a new hire feel appreciated by your department and the organization. You can even make the reward fun, such as a syringe-shaped highlighter for mastering the blood draw process or toy eyeglasses for seeing and fulfilling a need.

If it's close to a major holiday, invite a new hire who hasn't yet started to come in and participate in decorating the department. This is a great nonthreatening way to help the new nurse ease into the group, and it helps to build social connections.

Open the Feedback Door

Don't miss the opportunity to give your staff plenty of feedback, which is particularly important for Generation Y nurses who are used to receiving regular feedback and may feel isolated if you do not take the time to let them know how they are doing—even if it's just to say they are doing a great job.

You should hold formal evaluations at various stages during a new nurse's first year: Consider 30, 60, 90, and 120 days. But don't make these the only time you give feedback—give positive feedback all the time.

To coincide with a new staff members' 90-day evaluation—at which point they should be starting to feel like they have settled in and are on their way to being part of the team—give them a personalized card from your staff (or at least from all staff members on their shift and their peer mentors). You can get creative and personalize them even further by scanning in a picture of the team or a picture of the new employee in action during his or her orientation. Also, have everyone sign the card, and present it during a staff meeting. It's a small but meaningful way to tell your newest team members that they're welcome in your department, they're important, and you want them to be successful.

Another way to give positive affirmation is to send a handwritten note to an employee's family and/or spouse. As my 90-day evaluation approached, my supervisor mailed a card to my husband and me, and inside she included a note to my husband. She knew his name and included several compliments about my performance and thanked him for "loaning me" to the department for 40 hours a week. I cannot even begin to tell you how much that impressed both of us!

Invite new nurses who have been hired in the last 90 days to come to your office and have breakfast with you. This provides them the opportunity to share experiences, ideas, and thoughts about the profession.

Mentoring Programs Provide Vital Support

Encouraging mentoring relationships can be a key tool in aiding retention, particularly for new nurse graduates. Mentors help to inspire mentees, and as role models they also support and encourage mentees.

Throughout all aspects of nursing, mentorships offer approaches to creating close working partnerships between mentors and mentees as a vital element of the work experience. The most successful mentorships are those that are structured, one-to-one partnerships that focus on the professional and psychosocial needs of the mentee within the context of a collegial relationship. They foster caring and supportive interactions and encourage mentees to develop to their fullest potential.

Some of the roles mentors can fulfill with mentees include (Vance, 2000):

• Orient the new nurse to the unit

• Provide leadership, guidance, and emotional support

• Model and facilitate growth in professional behaviors and skills

• Encourage and facilitate stress management

• Give and receive constructive criticism and feedback on strengths and weaknesses with suggestions for improvement

• Teach how to handle new responsibilities and take acceptable risks

• Balance personal and professional commitments

• Listen and communicate with empathy, insight, and wisdom

- Provide professional and career-counseling information

- Follow through on all commitments

If you want to create a formal mentoring program, it's important to find people who will relate well to each other, and for both mentor and mentee to have a good understanding of what the relationship will involve and what the goals should be. The two tools following, Figures 4.2 and 4.3, can be used at the beginning of the relationship. The mentor application form helps establish goals, while answering the 10 questions in Figure 4.3 helps mentors and mentees become better acquainted. Once they have thoroughly answered the questions themselves, provide each individual with the other's answers.

Figure 4.2	Mentor Application Form

Name: _____ **Years of service:** _____

Service/routing symbol: _____ Phone number: _____

Current grade/position title: _____

Educational background: _____

_____

Occupational areas where you have experience that you are willing to share through a mentoring relationship: _____

_____

_____

Special knowledge/skills/experiences you are willing to share through a mentorship relationship (e.g., public speaking, office automation, professional organizations, education or volunteer programs, etc.): _____

_____

_____

What personal characteristics/abilities qualify you to serve as a mentor?

_____

_____

If selected, I agree to serve as a mentor for the Mentoring Program at the *Location*, *Address* (Contact person, phone).

Signature: _____ Date: _____

Supervisor's signature/concurrence (if applicable): _____

Date: _____

Complete and return this application form to: _____

Source: Diana Swihart, PhD, DMin, MSN,CS, RN-BC, clinical nurse specialist in nursing education at the Bay Pines VA Healthcare System in Bay Pines, FL. Adapted with permission.

| Figure 4.3 | **Mentor Relationship Guide** |

Mentor/mentee name: _____

Current position: _____ Location: _____

Phone: _____ Fax: _____

E-mail: _____

Describe your primary job activity: _____
_____
_____

What do you hope to gain from this mentoring relationship? _____
_____
_____

What do you bring to this mentoring relationship? _____
_____
_____

What non-nursing interests or hobbies do you have? _____
_____
_____

In what professional nursing organizations do you actively participate?
_____
_____

Which days, times, and how long would you like to meet with your mentor/mentee?
_____
_____

| Figure 4.3 | Mentor Relationship Guide (cont.) |

Would you prefer face-to-face meetings, telephone sessions, e-mail, other (explain)?

_____

_____

How would you prefer disagreements to be handled? _____

_____

_____

Describe the type of feedback you would prefer (e.g., verbal, written, or both)

_____

_____

Describe what role you would most like your mentor to play: advisor, coach, teacher, guide, resource person, etc. _____

_____

What questions do you have about your mentor/mentee? _____

_____

_____

Summary comments: _____

_____

_____

Mentor or mentee signature: _____

Date: _____

Complete and return this evaluation to: _____

Source: Diana Swihart, PhD, DMin, MSN,CS, RN-BC, clinical nurse specialist in nursing education at the Bay Pines VA Healthcare System in Bay Pines, FL. Adapted with permission.

RETENTION GEM: CASE STUDY

Get Your New Nurses Past the Hurdles

About 50% of the new nurses in the emergency department (ED) at The Robert Wood Johnson University Hospital in New Brunswick, NJ, a Level 1 trauma center, could not make it through the department's orientation program and left within a year. The new grads who left reported feelings of helplessness and a lack of adequate support and preparation.

To stop the revolving door of having to continually recruit new nurses, the ED wanted to find ways to help novice nurses through the rough start and build a desire to stay in the field. So the department created a new mentoring program to help staff transition and improve their education and development. Developed by Anthony Filippelli, BS, RN, CEN, head nurse in the ED, and Kathleen Evanovich Zavotsky, MS, RN, CCRN, CEN, APRN, BC, clinical nurse specialist, the department took off running with a program aptly titled "Be a Mentor, Not a Tormentor."

Beginning the process

Filipelli and Zavotsky decided the mentoring program would fill a vital missing step in the hospital's training program for new ED nurses.

"New grads kept asking for a mentoring program," says Zavotsky. "They felt a little leery about ending their orientation. They were done with orientation and boom, that was it. It was a little lacking."

The new program pairs nurses with a mentor after they have completed the original preceptor training program. The mentors, who volunteer their time, are nurses that have been at the hospital for at least three years and have ED experience.

RETENTION GEM: CASE STUDY

After deciding to become a mentor—defined in the program as "a colleague who is willing to guide, teach, and support during the growth of a novice's practice"—nurses fill out an application. Mentors then go through a training session, where they discuss the program and what it means to be a mentor. The group is taught a number of learning techniques to help new nurses navigate the waters in the ED.

There are 10 steps to being a good mentor:

1. Remember what it was like to be a novice

2. Acknowledge the presence of the new nurse

3. Openly discuss a plan

4. Remain with them through thick and thin

5. Assist them in critical thinking development

6. Provide them with insight into the chain of command

7. Remain positive

8. Remain aware of your influence and behave accordingly

9. Befriend them

10. Be a good listener

The mentors are given navy blue T-shirts with white letters that read "Mentor, Not a Tormentor." Each new nurse is paired with two mentors, which ensures that one mentor will be around each time the mentee works.

RETENTION GEM: CASE STUDY

For the first two weeks, the mentee follows the mentor's schedule within the department. During the first three months, the mentor and the mentee meet every two weeks to talk about everything, from educational opportunities within the field to any difficult cases either one has faced.

After three months, the pair start meeting every three weeks, which decreases to every month after six months. One of the biggest results of the program, says Filipelli, is that new nurses report not experiencing the nervousness and anxiety often associated with approaching an older nurse with questions—evidence that the techniques had accomplished the goal of ending horizontal hostility within the group.

Getting results

After the first year of the program, Filipelli says he retained 9 out of the 10 nurses involved with the program. The one nurse that left only did so because she was relocated to another trauma center, adds Filipelli.

Mentors and mentees complete evaluations, and Zavotsky says the feedback has been phenomenal. Most department nurses, she says, view the program as team-building and wish for it to continue.

"Mentees and mentors have nothing but positive things to say about it," she says. "I have so many people that want to be mentors now, much more than the [original] 13. Every time I hire a new person, they say, 'If you need a mentor, I'll be a mentor.'"

The need for mentors in any unit is crucial to nurse retention, says Filipelli, but with the exceptionally stressful atmosphere of an emergency unit, the need is especially strong.

RETENTION GEM: CASE STUDY

So how do I do it?

A mentoring program is not the type of program that takes a particularly long time to get up and running in a facility, says Filipelli, making it an effective, quick method to increase nurse retention and job satisfaction. He says he also believes that mentoring programs should be strictly voluntary.

Another piece of advice: don't get discouraged if the group starts off small. "If you could even get two or three on a voluntary basis for the first year, the next time around you would see that many more people want to do it," says Filipelli

Source: The Staff Educator, May 2007, HCPro, Inc. Adapted with permission.

Everyone needs a buddy

As well as formal mentor programs, there are many other types of supportive relationships that will help new graduate nurses make it through their difficult first year as a nurse. Some organizations assign new nurses a buddy to help them through the first days or weeks. A buddy can be someone to sit with in the lunchroom or a resource to ask day-to-day questions, such as how to get to another part of the hospital when they need to help transfer a patient.

Also introduce new graduate nurses with other new graduates in the organization so they can form their own support system. Everyone likes to hear from other people who are going through the same things they are, and such support systems can be outlets for stress and opportunities for learning.

Proven Pearls

Danbury Health Systems (DHS) has administrative assistants who volunteer their time to bring each new nurse up to speed on such basics as use of the telephone, navigating the facility and the unit, and security issues. Each new nurse also acquires a buddy after the first month on the job. A buddy is a peer in the department with no more than three years of experience who can still remember what it was like to be a newbie. Selected by the manager, a buddy facilitates integration of the new employee into the crowd for the first 30 days, helps figure out interdepartmental relations and politics, and creates a one-on-one friendship that helps each new grad feel at home on the unit.

—**Phyllis Zappala, senior vice president of HR at Danbury Health Systems in Danbury, CT**

Soak in the Knowledge

It is also helpful to offer structured educational programs for new graduates, which could be part of a preceptoring program or a longer-term nurse residency program. Develop specific courses based on topics new graduates identify they need. For example, many new graduates have limited exposure to chest tubes in school. If your unit cares for a patient population that uses chest tubes in their plan of care, you might consider setting up a small skills lab and using a few experienced staff nurses to provide one-on-one coaching. Other clinical topics to consider include acute stroke care, ventilator management, blood gas analysis, and postmortem care (including having an opportunity to talk about feelings and fears when caring for dying patients).

Mastering these skills will help new nurse graduates advance beyond the novice phase. And if you have a clinical ladder program, include a class to explain how it works and why it is valuable for professional growth.

Proven Pearls

During new graduate nurses' first year at Danbury Health Systems (DHS), they attend a quarterly forum as a way to get together with other new employees, have fun, share experiences, and learn from experts. Sponsored by the HR department, these mixers provide touch points at which new employees can reconnect, compare notes, and build relationships outside their own department. Each forum has a theme, such as "Ask Senior Management," "Let's Talk About Service Excellence at DHS," and "Let's Talk About Development at DHS." The last theme outlines on-the-job and extracurricular growth opportunities with testimonials from staff veterans.

—Phyllis Zappala, senior vice president of HR at Danbury Health Systems in Danbury, CT.

References

Newhouse, R.P., J.J. Hoffman, J. Suflita, et al. (2007). "Evaluating an innovative program to improve new nurse graduate socialization into the acute health care setting." *Nursing Administration Quarterly* 31, 50–60.

Swihart, D. (2007). *Nurse Preceptor Program Builder: Tools for a Successful Preceptor Program, Second Edition*. Marblehead, MA: HCPro, Inc.

Vance, C. (2000). "R+A+A: The secret formula for making communication and delegation easier." Video 4 in the *Moments of Excellence* video series. Minneapolis: Creative Health Care Management.

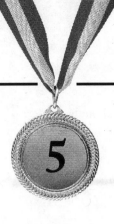

Be a Leader: Build Relationships, Promote Autonomy, and Listen to Nurses' Needs

Nurse-to-Manager Relationships

Numerous studies have published findings concluding that most employees leave their jobs due to unsatisfactory relationships with their manager. And when you talk to staff nurses about what makes them stay at their job, a common response is "my manager." Staff nurses are happy when they feel their manager respects their contributions and makes time for them. All nurse managers must develop an understanding of staff perceptions and how staff members relate their importance in the overall picture to how much time their manager spends with them.

Question yourself

Sometimes the best retention tool is to invest some time and money into refreshing and expanding your management skills repertoire. Do a quick personal analysis and honestly answer these questions:

- Do I have an open-door policy or is it dependent on the events of the day?

- Am I giving clear expectations for each staff member or is there room to offer more details?

- Am I giving timely annual evaluations and noting more areas of strength than areas that need improvement?

- Am I on time for scheduled meetings with my staff?

- Are our staff meetings more about what's wrong than celebrating what's right?

- Am I encouraging my staff toward professional growth and providing a way for staff members to advance?

- Do my staff members have the tools and equipment they need to provide excellent care?

Proven Pearls

The manager is the key in nurse retention and the manager must have leadership support from above. The manager must have the usual managerial attributes: consistency, fairness, advocacy, good listening skills, and strong communication skills. Other attributes I have tried to incorporate into my management style include honesty, family-oriented, valuing personal relationships with my staff, professional growth and values, fostering and maintaining projects, and staying dedicated to change.

—Patricia Crabtree, RN, BSN, MHA, CNA, nurse manager at Saint Joseph Hospital in Atlanta

Have a heart

Sometimes the easiest way to recognize your nursing staff is to show you care by having an open-door policy or just asking how their day is going. Try these seven tips and see what a difference you can make:

1. Schedule to meet with a different staff person one day per week for coffee or sit with him or her at lunch time. Preschedule and post this information so staff members can look forward to it.

2. Post dates and times when you will have an "open door" for anyone who needs to talk.

3. Be available at shift changes several times per week.

4. Rotate the staff from each shift to participate in hiring interviews. Schedule new-hire interviews to be convenient for the staff you currently have instead of the applicants. There is no better way to build a team than to teach the staff that you currently have to be involved in the hiring process.

5. Arrange coverage for a staff person for an hour or two, and take him or her with you to one of your management meetings (e.g., department head or a council). This not only allows the staff person a glimpse into what management does all day, but it also shows that you believe in his or her ability to handle increased responsibility. Take a different staff member each month.

6. Hand out paychecks instead of sticking them in a drawer to be picked up. Even in an open-door atmosphere, some employees will never speak up. Handing out paychecks ensures that at least once per month (or however often you choose to do it) every staff person will have an opportunity to ask a question, voice a concern, or suggest an idea.

7. Consider a staff brainstorming event to formulate a unit mission that describes the care philosophy of your department for your patient population. Giving staff members an opportunity to be a part of developing your unit mission will help them feel engaged. You can refer back to the mission statement they developed when confronted with resistance during implementation of required changes.

Have the unit mission printed on a plaque or mural and hang it prominently in your department.

Proven Pearls

I find the relationship as important as the job. The process entails listening, service on my part, attention to their time-off needs (even if it interferes with mine), equal recognition, and thanks in front of peers when justified. Be there for your nurses in every way. A nurse needs backup, from a blown light bulb to securing whatever is needed for patient care to continue. My job is to get out of the way and remove the barriers so they can be effective. Always look for the bright side and keep your sense of humor. In the end, learn to say "I'm sorry, there's no quick fix, but I'm not leaving you with the problem."

—**Beverly Loscher, RN, long-term care director of nursing
at TLC Health Nursing Facility in Irving, NY**

Be detail-oriented

To help build a strong relationship with your nurses use a variety of tips from this book. But it can be hard to remember everything in your busy day, so create a calendar to remember birthdays, anniversaries, graduations, and even days when you can let your CNO know all the accomplishments your staff members have achieved. After you have created your calendar (see Figure 5.1), remember to do the following:

- Send out electronic cards by using free Web sites:

    – *www.123greetings.com*   – *www.yahoo.americangreetings.com*

    – *www.bluemountain.com*   – *www.fun-greetings-jokes.com*

    – *www.hallmark.com*   – *www.regards.com*

    – *www.free-e-cards-online.com*   – *www.care2.com*

    – *www.greetingsnecards.com*   – *www.christianet.com*

    – *www.egreetings.com*   – *http://reminders.barnesandnoble.com*

    – *www.dayspring.com*   – *www.higreetings.com*

- Recount nurses' contributions for the year in their anniversary card and describe specific ways they are important to your unit. This goes beyond the standard listing of goals attained on their annual evaluation—it shows your appreciation for each nurse's unique efforts toward the success of the organization.

- Know nurses' favorite things, such as candy, hobbies, food, and even music. Keep an alphabetical file of the "favorites" list (see Figure 5.2) for each staff member and retrieve information for those spontaneous rewards.

Figure 5.1 **Calendar**

May

Sun	Mon	Tue	Wed	Thu	Fri	Sat
				1 *Send birthday cards*	2	3
4	5 *Reward two nurses with movie tickets or coffee coupon*	6	7	8	9	10
11	12	13	14 *Post a thank you note on unit for all staff to see*	15	16	17
18	19 *Have a unit pizza party*	20	21	22	23 *Record nurses' accomplishments in their ongoing performance development records*	24
25	26	27 *Update CNO with all the great work staff nurses have completed for the month*	28	29	30	31

Proven Pearls

You have to get personal with your staff and develop a sense of family. Your unit becomes a "home away from home." Although this is work, it is okay to have fun. Develop social bonds with each other. Have parties for special events (at work and outside work). The relationships among the staff on this unit go far beyond work. We get involved with each other during bad times. We've supported each other during financial crises, divorce, illness, and death. We also celebrate weddings, babies, graduations, and birthdays. The staff needs to feel part of the group, and they must be recognized.

—**Patricia Crabtree, RN, BSN, MHA, CNA, nurse manager at Saint Joseph Hospital in Atlanta**

Figure 5.2	Sample Employee "Favorites" List

Keep an alphabetical file of the "favorites" list for all staff and retrieve information for those spontaneous rewards!

Please list your favorite:

Color: _____

Hobby: _____

Snack food: _____

Candy: _____

Meal: _____

Sport: _____

Type of music: _____

Reading material: _____

What size socks do you wear: _____

Do you have a CD player in your car: _____

Source: Shelley Cohen, RN, BS, CEN, founder and president of Health Resources Unlimited, www.hru.net, in Tennessee. Reprinted with permission.

Staff Schedules to Please All Generations

Dissatisfaction with the scheduling process is a major bone of contention at many organizations. Trying to make a schedule that keeps all nurses happy is not easy when there are four generations in our work force today, as discussed in detail in Chapter 3. These generations are:

- Silent generation: born 1926–1946

- Baby boomers: born 1947–1962

- Generation X: born 1963–1979

- Generation Y: born in 1980 and thereafter

As a manager, you just want the shifts filled with an adequate blend of new and seasoned nurses to provide safe, quality, competent, and compassionate care to patients. With careful planning and ongoing dialogue, you can create a schedule that will please all generations.

Stop! Don't let the silent generation leave

Offer the experienced nurses the following options to help them work at a pace that is comfortable for them:

- **Eight-hour schedules:** Many silents would like an opportunity to return to eight-hour shifts, especially if they work in a physically demanding unit.

- **Multitask scheduling:** Schedule a 12-hour shift that contains several tasks. For example, they could first work a four-hour physical patient care assignment, then a less physical four-hour period (e.g., a mentoring role), and then another four-hour physical patient care assignment.

- **Peak-time scheduling:** Create peak-time shifts (e.g., four to six hours per day, five days per week). This allows silents to work hours that suit them while providing the unit with valuable relief at busy times.

- **Combined schedules:** Allow the silents to band together as a group to create their own eight-hour schedules. They can jointly sign up for eight-hour shifts, but they must match each other to cover a full 24 hours so there is no negative effect on others. This can be an especially good option for weekend shifts when the staffing numbers are usually lower.

Be flexible to baby boomers and Generation X

These two generations enjoy flexibility with their schedules, so consider these options:

- **Concurrent shifts:** Some nurses want all of their days concurrently, with long stretches off, so allow them the option of working 12-hour shifts and the opportunity to self-schedule within the structure of unit guidelines.

- **Staggered shifts:** Some nurses do not want to work more than two 12-hour shifts in a row. Offer them the option of two 12-hour shifts and two eight-hour shifts, which gives them three days off per week and five evenings off to be with family or friends, creating a work-life balance they appreciate.

You can do it Generation Y!

This generation sometimes lacks the stamina to withstand the demands of 12-hour shifts, but their biggest problem may be adapting to the loss of time with family or friends. They need understanding and guidance to make this work.

If your unit allows self-scheduling, this can be a powerful tool to keep this generation happy. Self-scheduling allows them input and control over their schedule.

Be sure to provide insight over Generation Y nurses when they begin to self-schedule. They may need assistance to ensure that they get the right balance and career development opportunities.

Proven Pearls

My unit is a 32-bed telemetry/step-down unit with approximately 80 very diverse employees, and it took several months for me to build trust among all of these employees.

One of the biggest hurdles on this unit was scheduling and staffing. I have a mixture of full-time, part-time, per diem, and weekend care. Staff members were sending me schedules that did not meet the requirements of their work agreement or their per diem contracts. Thus, the first thing I did was put out the work schedule for my full- and part-time staff to fill in their hours, and then I put out a schedule for the per diem contingent staff to fill in the open hours that were needed. This caused quite an upheaval, but eventually it worked out.

I put together four RNs to make a scheduling committee and had them write guidelines for scheduling, which included specifics about meeting weekend commitments and holidays. The overtime list that comes out after the schedule list has a rule stating that you can sign up for overtime only if you have not called in on a previous schedule. The other thing I did in relation to this was assign two RN schedulers on the unit—one for the day shift and one for the night shift. They are responsible for putting out the draft and entering the schedule. This has moved the responsibility of following the scheduling guidelines to the staff nurse and holding him or her accountable.

—Donna Noe, clinical manager of 2 East at Huron Valley Sinai Hospital in Commerce Township, MI

Proven Pearls

We actively work on respect with our staff. We realize they have a life beyond this place and encourage them to enjoy it. We have self-scheduling in the truest sense. One of our unit nurses is responsible for going over the schedule and making sure we do not have too many on one shift and not enough on another and [that] holidays are covered and so forth. We give nurses autonomy to make things better for the patients and for themselves.

—**Charlene Gordon, RN, clinical coordinator, ER emergency preparedness manager at Huntsville Memorial Hospital in Huntsville, AL**

Keep An Open Ear

A simple way to find out what motivates your staff—and crucially what will make them stay—is to ask them. You want to keep a finger on the pulse of why they are leaving, but more importantly, why they are staying.

What did you say?

Periodically ask different members of your team, "What do you like about working on this unit?" Continue to build upon the things they note. If they cannot think of anything, you have some work to do.

Take a look at the retention survey (see Figure 5.3) to get an understanding of how to improve nurse retention.

Figure 5.3	Retention Survey

1. Name one thing that you wish your manager did or offered to you.

2. If you could name one thing the organization could offer you as an employee, what would it be?

3. Can you name two things we offer you that keep you here as an employee?

4. What do you think are the two most common reasons people leave our department/organization?

5. Which of the following would be an important benefit for you/your family?

   • Pick up/drop off dry cleaning

   • Packaged complete dinners one night a week for a discounted price at local store

   • Car wash discount card

   • On-site banking

6. Is there anything in particular about this organization that makes you feel proud to be an employee here?

7. If you could change one thing that you think would have the greatest impact on improving retention, what would it be?

8. Name one thing a coworker recently did that made you feel valued as an employee.

9. Name one thing your manager has done to make you feel valued as an employee.

10. Share something a previous employer did that you felt had an impact on retention.

11. What have you heard from other nurses outside of our organization that impacts their retention?

Source: Shelley Cohen, RN, BS, CEN, founder and president of Health Resources Unlimited, www.hru.net, in Tennessee. Reprinted with permission.

Gauge the satisfaction meter

To really know to what extent nurses feel they are valuable to the organization, give them a nursing satisfaction survey (see Figure 5.4) where they can reveal their thoughts. Share the survey results with nursing leadership and your recruitment/ retention committee. This will help leadership celebrate their success areas and develop action plans for their problem areas.

You should conduct the nursing satisfaction survey on an annual basis to keep your finger on the pulse of your nursing staff. The survey should:

- Either include all levels of the nursing staff (RNs, licensed practical nurses, student nurses, certified nursing assistants, etc.), or the surveys can be RN-specific

- Benchmark its results against other similar facilities and units and compare the results with other units within the organization

Figure 5.4 **Nursing Satisfaction Questions**

Sample questions to ask:

1. What do you like best about your unit? The organization?

2. What do you like least about your unit? The organization?

3. Do you feel supported by your coworkers? Your management? If not, why not?

4. Are you provided with opportunities to improve your skills and grow professionally?

5. Is your unit adequately staffed with nursing staff? Support staff?

6. Does your unit have good morale?

7. Do you feel that the organization has a good benefits plan?

8. Do you feel that the organization's pay structure is competitive in the local market?

9. Do you feel that your unit offers flexible scheduling options?

10. Are you pleased with the amount of recognition that you receive for a job well done?

11. Would you recommend your unit and the organization to others?

Lydia Ostermeier, MSN, RN, CHCR, Clarian Health Partners. Reprinted with permission.

Pay Attention to the Beginning and the End

One of the best retention tips is to ensure that you're hiring the right staff from the very beginning. Sometimes we may not be asking the correct questions in the initial interview. Here are seven questions that you can use to gain particular insight:

1. "Tell me about a time when you had to adjust to another nurse or nurse assistant's working style to provide excellent patient care."

2. "Can you give me an example of a time when you set a goal and were able to meet or achieve it? What obstacles did you have to work through along the way?"

3. "Can you give me a specific example of a time when you used good judgment and logic in solving a complex patient or family situation?"

4. "What is the most creative thing you have done in a clinical position?"

5. "What was the last continuing education seminar you attended?"

6. "Are you a member of any professional nursing organizations?"

7. "Please tell me about the most beneficial nursing seminar you have attended."

Check their pulse—they may have retention tips

Exit interviews are extremely important because you want to get a reading on the reasons people are leaving. If possible, it is beneficial to have someone else conduct the exit interview, such as a nurse recruiter or someone in human resources. You will most likely have a few unit-specific questions to ask, but be sure to include some variation of these:

• Please tell me two things you would change tomorrow if you were the manager of this unit.

- If you could change one thing about this organization, what would it be?

- What one thing would have prevented you from looking for a new position?

- What about your job satisfied you the most?

- What about your job was the least satisfying to you?

- What does your new job offer you that we were unable to provide?

Reference

Lower, J. (2006). *A Practical Guide to Managing the Multigenerational Workforce: Skills for Nurse Managers.* Marblehead, MA: HCPro, Inc.

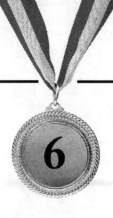

Team Building: The Road to a Positive Work Environment

The Link: Happier Nurses Equal Better Outcomes

Do happy nurses have better patient outcomes? Research shows that positive work environments are directly linked with better patient satisfaction scores, improved patient safety, and great overall recruitment and retention (AONE, 2003). Lots of attention has been given to unhealthy work environments contributing to staff burnout, disengagement, and turnover. So, how do you shift the paradigm and turn a unit that has a lot of negativity and low satisfaction into a greater-performing unit with a healthy work environment? The answer may be by focusing on one nurse at a time and turning those individuals into a team. This chapter will discuss ways to promote a cohesive team environment on your unit and help your nurses feel like they work in a supportive environment.

Nurse managers set the tone

If an organization has one or more problem units that are experiencing less-than-optimal outcomes, nursing leadership should assess the effectiveness of the clinical managers of those units. Nurse managers can be viewed as the "chief retention officers" for their clinical areas, and as discussed previously, one of the key reasons nursing staff members give for leaving an organization is their relationship with their clinical managers.

Nurse managers set the tone for the whole unit. It is one of the most difficult jobs in the nursing organization, but it is also one of the most rewarding. If you are not fully engaged with your staff and with workplace issues, the environment can quickly deteriorate. Clinical managers must have great interpersonal and organizational skills, resiliency to hold staff members accountable, integrity, and they must be accessible to the staff. In a lot of organizations, managers are pulled further and further away from their clinical units due to their participation in multiple meetings and committees, and therefore they are less accessible to their staff, physicians, and the patients they serve. If a unit starts to experience turnover and dissatisfied staff members, it is time to reassess where that unit's manager is spending his or her time. You must invest in your staff to get the best outcome you desire.

A Relationship-Building Culture

Engaging with the staff is a key to retention, but it's also important to help staff members feel engaged with each other. Staff members do not have to be best friends, but they do have to form collaborative, supportive, respectful relationships with each other. Another reason nurses leave an organization, besides their relationship with their nurse manager, is their relationship with their coworkers. It is vital to get to know one another as a team and as individuals. This can be much easier if you help to create opportunities for staff members to form relationships.

Form a celebration committee

One way to build relationships—and to take all of the responsibility for ideas off your shoulders!—is to form a celebration committee on the unit.

The celebration committee can assume many different functions. The committee might plan monthly or quarterly celebration activities that appeal to all ages and genders, such as cookouts, sports outings, or picnics. Again, whatever the group can do to encourage growth of personal relationships within the team will contribute to staff retention and an improved positive workplace.

The celebration committee can also plan the yearly holiday party, which is usually the ultimate challenge. It can be difficult to execute a celebration that will meet the needs of your staff, particularly while working with a (usually) tight budget. The committee will first need to consult with you, the nurse manager, to attain a budget figure. Then, they need to pick a date and a venue. They should be creative with planning and make sure the event appeals to all staff members: holiday party formats can include bowling, a nice dinner, theatre tickets, a simple potluck luncheon or dinner with ample time to sit and chat.

Ensure that as many staff members as possible can attend the party by suggesting that a sister unit help with staffing or by allowing casual hourly or supplemental staff members to work the date and time of the event.

Collect praise

Boost morale when nurses reach the "oversaturated" stage by having everyone write on pieces of paper one compliment or one thing they admire about their peers. Collect the papers and distribute them to the staff. You can conduct this during staff meetings, while walking rounds during a shift, or by posting a memo on the unit bulletin board. Encourage nurses to keep their "notes" in a folder or book as an instant way to boost morale on days when they are feeling down and need to know how their team feels about them. Figure 6.1 is an example of a sheet you can distribute to nurses.

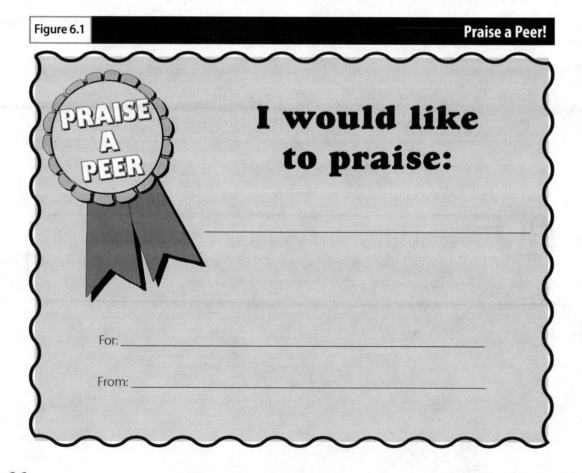

Figure 6.1 — **Praise a Peer!**

PRAISE A PEER

I would like to praise:

_____

For: _____

From: _____

Nurse Retention Toolkit

Age is only a number

Get a multigenerational group together and start talking about the defining moments in their lives. This is a great way for multigenerational groups to establish relationships and bonding. Stimulate the discussion by asking questions such as (Martin, 2004):

1. What was cool when you were growing up?

2. What was all the rage in fashion?

3. What music and movies did you like growing up?

4. Who were your role models?

5. What is important to your generation?

6. What are your core values?

The Perfect Getaway: A Nursing Retreat

A very effective team-building strategy is to get away from the hospital and hold a team retreat. This can sound like an impossible endeavor, but the benefits from the event can offset the financial and organizational challenges.

Warning: Hospital scrubs not allowed

An off-site team retreat can boost morale and build a positive workplace. Optimally, this retreat will occur off-site twice a year to catch as many staff members as possible. Some good venues for retreats can be a clubhouse at an apartment building, a restaurant banquet hall, a nature center, or even a willing volunteer's house. The retreat can be a full day or a half day and can focus on numerous team-building exercises, or it can be a mix of some strategic planning with team-building activities interspersed throughout the day. The main purpose is to promote team spirit by getting to know other team members on a more personal basis.

It is important during the team-building retreat to reward and recognize the nursing staff. This is a great chance to celebrate accomplishments and work efforts that routinely go unnoticed. Another important factor is to ensure that the team is split into groups that don't already have a working relationship when conducting small group activities. This will ensure that groups of individuals will get to know others in their team that they don't traditionally work with, thus further fostering team spirit and camaraderie. Figure 6.2 is an example agenda for a team-building retreat.

Figure 6.2	Team-Building Retreat Agenda
May 7	
8:30 a.m. – 8:45 a.m	Coffee, tea, and soft drinks
8:45 a.m. – 9 a.m.	Welcome from nurse manager and CNO
9 a.m. – 10 a.m.	Get to know your colleagues better with human bingo!
10 a.m. – 10:30 a.m.	Set yearly goals
10:30 a.m. – 10:45 a.m.	Break with snacks
10:45 a.m. – 11:45 a.m.	Nursing rewards and recognition
11:45 a.m. – 12:30 p.m.	Nurses share accomplishments and nursing best practices
12:30 p.m. – 1:30 p.m.	Lunch
1:30 p.m. – 3 p.m.	Discuss the team's strong points, areas for improvement, and how to become a stronger team
3 p.m. – 3:15 p.m.	Break with snacks
3:15 p.m. – 4:15 p.m.	Play games!

Proven Pearls

Play human bingo during staff meetings by creating a bingo card that features squares describing certain characteristics or preferences of staff members. The descriptions should be unrelated to work (e.g., favorite color is purple, rides a motorcycle, enjoys vacationing in Mexico). Have the staff nurses take five minutes at the beginning of the meeting to get as many squares signed as possible with the correct members' names; the first member who shouts "bingo!" ends the activity. To get the group interacting even more, have the bingo winner share a few of the signatures in the squares.

—**Michele Wilmoth, BSN, RN, Magnet Recognition Program®**
coordinator at Akron Children's Hospital in Akron, OH

To set goals for areas that need improvement, see Figure 6.3—a team assessment in which nurses can rate different characteristics and qualities of the team, and then summarize strengths and weaknesses so leadership can develop an action plan to address these areas for improvement.

| Figure 6.3 | **Team Assessment** |

Use the following assessment to rate your team members. Rate the team as you view it today with 5 being exceptional and 1 being consistently deficient. Circle your response.

1. Every team member has a clear idea of the team's goals.   1 2 3 4 5

2. All team members respect each other.   1 2 3 4 5

3. The team communicates openly.   1 2 3 4 5

4. The team members resolve conflict/disagreements.   1 2 3 4 5

5. The team members support each other.   1 2 3 4 5

6. The team members support leadership.   1 2 3 4 5

7. There is opportunity for input into decisions.   1 2 3 4 5

8. Team members get encouragement for new ideas.   1 2 3 4 5

9. Team members freely express their real views.   1 2 3 4 5

10. There is little negativity among team members.   1 2 3 4 5

Please answer in full sentences the following questions:

What are our team's strong points (i.e., what are we doing well)? _____

_____

What do we need to focus on for improvement? _____

_____

What suggestions do you have to make us a stronger team? _____

_____

Source: Lydia Ostermeier, MSN, RN, CHCR, Clarian Health in Indianapolis, IN. Adapted with permission.

Examples of suggestions to build a stronger team include:

- Building stronger communication and trust

- Having lunch with a team member you don't usually hang out with

- Being more open to change

- Forgiving and moving on after differences

- Creating a more efficient way to give negative feedback

- Having a clear understanding of his or her position, but allowing others to pitch in and help when it's needed

- Developing goals and a mission statement for the team

Ready, set, game time!

Games are a fun way to break the ice, conduct discussions, and promote nursing education.

One game to try is hot potato, which focuses on rapid-fire answers to questions related to nursing. To start, use a ball in place of the hot potato and have employees sit in a circle. A nurse manager should ask a question to the group, set a timer for 60 seconds, and toss the potato to one person, who will then quickly try to answer the question and then toss the potato to someone else. Once the next player has caught the potato, ask another question.

The object of the game is to not get stuck with the hot potato when time runs out. Players get rid of the hot potato by answering questions correctly. If the time runs out while a player has the hot potato, he or she is eliminated from the game.

Remember spelling bees from your school days? The bee game will help participants learn nursing facts and other valuable material. And remember, the goal is to be the last one standing.

Have the participants stand in line across the front of a meeting room or the cafeteria. A host (e.g., a representative from leadership) asks each participant one question at a time. If a participant answers correctly, he or she goes to the end of the line. If a participant answers incorrectly, he or she is eliminated. The host then asks a question of the next participant. The host continues asking questions until only one person, who has answered all of his or her questions correctly, is left standing. That person is known as the Bee Queen or Bee King. Reward the winner with a prize, such as a large jar of honey—a suitable award for winning this title.

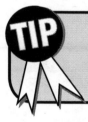

Turn this into a tournament by having the bee winners compete in an organizationwide contest. Post the photos of each department's winners in the cafeteria or on the intranet.

Caution: Nurses at work

Team building doesn't have to take place at a fancy location with a set agenda. One hospital shows that it can take place within the community by trading scrubs for hard hats.

Proven Pearls

Mercy General Health Partners in Muskegon, MI, recently merged with Hackley Hospital to form Mercy Health Partners. During the merger process, nurses from both organizations teamed up to focus on serving their community by sponsoring a Habitat for Humanity house. A committee of staff nurses worked with Habitat for Humanity to coordinate fundraising efforts and volunteers to raise the $40,000 and labor necessary to build the house. The nursing group chose the name "Muskegon Nurses Care" to portray the partnership and mission of the project. To raise money, staff nurses have teamed together and focused on the following fundraising efforts:

- Selling T-shirts with the Muskegon Nurses Care logo
- Hosting an omelet buffet and a silent auction at a local country club (all auction items were donated)
- Soliciting individual contributions through a mailing to all Mercy Health Partners employees
- Holding events focusing on scrapbooking, a barbeque chicken dinner, and a wine and cheese party
- Selling ball caps, visors, and water bottles with the Muskegon Nurses Care logo

—**Kathy Breunsbach, RN, special projects coordinator at Mercy Health Partners in Muskegon, MI**

Nurse-to-Nurse Communication

Build communication and improve team-building efforts by encouraging nurses to talk about their achievements, or about instances when they were challenged by a difficult patient care assignment and how they handled the situation. This provides dialogue on best practices to handle difficult patients to improve patient care.

Fill a room with chatter

Staff meetings are a great time to begin successful team building by putting three components in place:

1. Goal-oriented tasks developed by the team members with the mission of the organization in mind

2. The establishment of team roles defining the process in which the members will work together

3. The assessment of resources such as time, budgeting, educational tools, and administrative support

Once these components are in place, the team can begin to facilitate the group work by seeking input from each member, agreeing on a timetable for tasks, providing guidance, and helping members overcome barriers. Team norms should be taken into account and should consist of acceptable standards of behavior within the group, such as listening, talking, meeting agendas, and managing time.

Sustaining team effectiveness is necessary to achieve the expected end results. This can be accomplished through:

• Clearly stated visions and goals

• Distributed leadership

• Sharing of the workload

• A social environment that is open, is supportive, and focuses on learning

Promote talking across the organization

Most organizations host periodic employee forums during which upcoming changes or a "state of the organization" presentation is given. But this can also work well at the unit level. Many units are grouped in clusters (e.g., maternal/child health; critical care; med-surg). Consider getting these cluster units together in a forum to discuss organizational goals. You could have a few different focus groups work on interdepartmental goals ahead of time and either present their findings or solicit peer feedback. If you have a shared governance structure, it could provide an excellent avenue through which to facilitate this type of intervention.

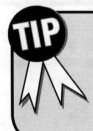

Once goals are established, consider a small giveaway item as a reminder of your goals. For example, a toy version of a compass could symbolize "We are headed in the direction of achieving 90% in patient satisfaction scores." Set realistic and achievable goals that staff members can envision and on which they can work together to feel a part of the organization.

References

American Organization of Nurse Executives (AONE). (2003.) *Healthy Work Environments: Striving for Excellence*, Volume II, AONE. Washington, DC.

Martin, C.A. (2004.) "Bridging the generation gap." *Nursing* 34 (12): 62-63.

Part 3

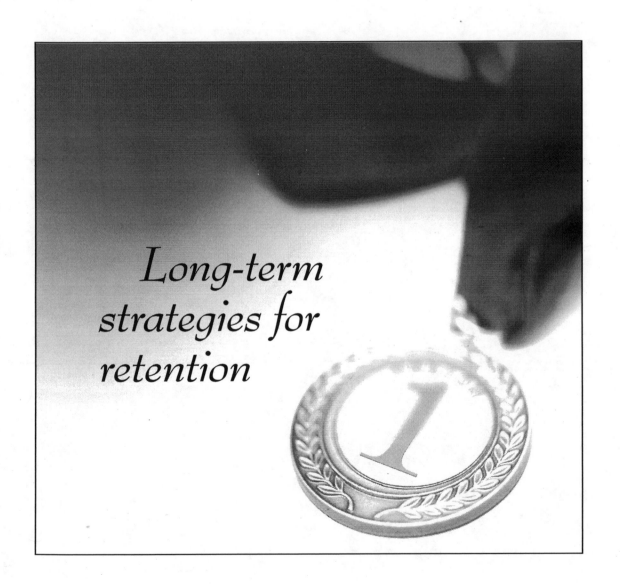

Long-term strategies for retention

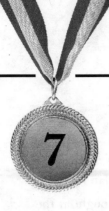

Build a Retention Budget

7

Managers Should Have a Retention Budget

The words *nurse* and *budget* typically are not mentioned in the same sentence. Budgeting and finance are frequently not taught in nursing school or in nursing orientation. But once you become a clinical manager, you are expected to be able to plan and execute many kinds of budgets, and one of them should be a retention budget. Retention budgets are necessary for implementing low-cost recognition and reward ideas that keep nurses happy, and for the expenditures that go along with improving professional development skills. As a manager, establishing a yearly budget will give you the tools you need to keep your nurses at the bedside.

Steps for Creating a Budget

As healthcare budgets get tighter, managers must become increasingly financially savvy for their organizations to survive. Thus, you must forecast and plan for the money that you need and then continually monitor your spending throughout the year so you come within budget at year's end.

Step 1: Research

When developing a retention budget, it is mandatory that you do some research beforehand. You must obtain much-needed data prior to the budget process so you can make calculated decisions as you form the budget framework. Once you have assembled your information, you can put the financial numbers together to help with strategic planning. The information you need for this includes:

- A strategic plan for retention activities

- The department's budget for the preceding calendar year

- Year-to-date monthly operating statements

- A list of major purchases that need to be made in the next calendar year

- Potential unit-based program expansions

Step 2: Create a strategic plan

Now craft a yearly retention strategic plan to help you accurately forecast, plan, and budget the dollars needed for retention activities. It takes a little coordination and collaboration with the human resources department, but the results can definitely be well worth the time spent. See Figure 7.1 for the nursing retention strategic plan that Clarian Health in Indianapolis put together.

Figure 7.1	Retention Strategic Plan

Unit/Cost center	Retention strategies
3 South Med-Surg	1. Implement unit clinical practice council 2. Implement unit celebration committee
SICU Critical Care	1. Construct healing sanctuary on unit to promote self-care 　of staff 2. Conduct grief workshop
PICU Peds Critical Care	1. Implement clinical advisor role on unit to help with on- 　boarding of new staff 2. Encourage 100% participation of staff in Healing Healthcare 　offering
BMTU Oncology	1. Involve staff with unit expansion development 2. Build travel money into the unit budget to allow staff to 　attend national conferences

Source: Lydia Ostermeier, MSN, RN, CHCR, Clarian Health in Indianapolis, IN. Adapted with permission.

Obtain Buy-In from Upper Management

How do you get upper management to listen to your requests for dollars to build a retention budget? You build a case.

Give nurses a voice

Set up a focus group with nurses to hear what retention efforts are important to them. You may be surprised by what they say because what you think is important may not be important to them. After the focus group, compile all the data, review it, and then come up with a wish list of the top 10 retention initiatives that were mentioned. Examples of unit-based retention efforts could be:

- On-site nursing conferences

- Reimbursement for certification

- Lift team labor and equipment

Once you have the wish list, prioritize it and allocate costs to each item. See Figure 7.2 for an example of a unit-based retention budget planning worksheet.

Figure 7.2	Retention Budget Planning Worksheet	

Item	Amount	Date needed/Goal
Specialty certifications		
Tuition reimbursement		
Continuing education		
Manager resource library		
Leadership development training		
Database development training		
Use of independent agency for exit interviewing		
Financial incentives for mentors		
Personal incentives programs (dry cleaning pick-up service, movie theatre tickets, exercise/gym memberships, etc.)		
Salary for retention		
Discounts for local vendors		
Nurses Week activities		
Funds to use for spontaneous rewards		
Annual recognition event with dinner, awards, and guest speaker		
Quarterly surprise events for all shifts that includes food and items from favorites list		

Source: Shelley Cohen, RN, BS, CEN, Health Resources Unlimited, www.hru.net. Reprinted with permission.

Get business savvy

Put together a strong business plan with an executive summary, associated budget, and any cost avoidance that could occur if the new program for each retention initiative is proposed. From here, take your proposal forward to upper management for consideration. Be prepared that the management team may not understand your needs, which is why it's important to have done research and written a proposal that explains how this will benefit the organization and retain nurses at the bedside.

The following discussion points should be included in a business plan for starting a lift team to help decrease nursing turnover. Internal drivers that are making a lift team a business necessity include:

- The loss of experienced workers

- Rising costs for employers (workers' compensation, restricted days, replacement workers to backfill positions, absenteeism)

- An increase in the morbidly obese patient population

Ideas for improvement include:

- Implementing a "no lift" standard of practice for nursing and assistive staff members

- Implementing a lift team in the hospital with 24/7 coverage

- Purchasing sufficient lift equipment and providing educational support and practice in its proper use

Once you state the internal drivers and ideas for improvement, determine projected costs for the lift team and equipment that you would like to purchase, and then end with the return on investment. Can cost avoidance be achieved by implementing your suggestions? Is what you suggested really worth it? Be sure to include the average cost for lost/restricted days for an RN in the past year and the orientation/ training replacement cost per RN. You can work with your employee occupational health and human resources to get these costs for your proposal.

Before you present your business case to the executives for approval, try to gain key stakeholder support for your proposal. Take these stakeholders for a cup of coffee, and discuss the key points of the proposal and allow them time to ask questions. Then, take your proposal forward for consideration. Always remember that the last step in budget preparation of any sort involves negotiating and compromising. You may not always get what you want the first time, but keep trying and emphasize the need as a retention effort.

The Other "R": Recruitment

Although it's vitally important to retain staff members, sometimes a position needs to be filled. For those times, meet with your in-house recruiter if you have one, or with human resources, to put together a plan on how you will approach hiring. Keep your recruitment budget in mind as you build a retention budget.

Look through the crystal ball

Be prepared to fill open nursing positions by forecasting your needs. Calculate the total number of RNs that need to be recruited and project how many will come from internal transfers versus external hires. This will help to predict orientation costs as internal transfers typically take less time to orient than external hires. Then, after you have decided how many hires will need to be recruited externally, develop tactical recruitment strategies with human resources or the recruiter that are going to be used to reach the target recruits.

Even though a strategic plan can help with forecasting costs for RNs, you must not forget to plan for any other position for which you might need to recruit. Do you typically need to recruit two unit secretaries and one equipment tech per year? Are these candidates available in the local market? Are you going to be expanding any programs that will require any new positions? When will you need these positions filled? You will need to ask all of these questions to accurately forecast your needs.

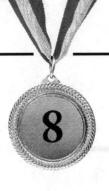

Take It to the Next Level: Advance Nursing Professional Development

Support Nursing Professional Development

It's important for nurses to advance their professional skills to meet the challenges of a changing work environment and improve bedside care to increase patient satisfaction and quality outcomes. But it's also important for healthcare organizations and nurse managers to have an infrastructure in place to support their nurses' professional development.

But how do you, as a nurse manager, support your nursing staff with tools to advance professionally? The opportunities to advance and recognize nurses' professional development skills are limitless whether your budget is small, large, or nonexistent.

Career Advancement Opportunities

Continuing education offers opportunity for nurses to grow in their profession and remain personally and professionally challenged. You can employ many strategies to encourage nursing staff members to return to school or attain certification in their clinical specialty.

Pack the bags—it's back to school time

It is important to assess the current educational demographics of your nursing staff to see what kinds of programs are needed. Are most of your staff members BSN-prepared? If so, perhaps all your organization may need is a nursing master's partnership. Do you have a large population of licensed practical nurses (LPNs)/licensed vocational nurses (LVNs)? Perhaps you could partner with a local RN program to provide these nurses an opportunity to get back to school.

We all know that going back to school is a huge sacrifice, as it takes time, effort, and most of all, money. If most of the nurses on your staff work full-time and have a family, returning to school may be low on their priority list. This is where establishing formal partnerships with nursing schools to bring degree programs on-site for professional staff members is important.

Clarian Health in Indianapolis formed a partnership with the University of Indianapolis in which the university brings instructors on-site to educate nurses. Both the BSN completion program and the MSN program meet one day per week for three to six hours throughout the course of study (usually three years for both degrees). This allows students to work with their supervisor to have that same day off over a period of time. This also improves managers' ability to plan for staffing and allows greater support for students.

In addition, the university has taken care of streamlining the admissions and registration processes, which is a huge satisfier for nurses. Clarian has worked out a process with the university to defer tuition fees until the end of the semester so the organization's tuition reimbursement policy can pick up the cost. This means no out-of-pocket tuition costs for the students. Furthermore, the university has created a way for students to order books for each class online and have them shipped directly to their homes.

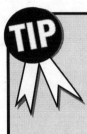

In the midst of nurses advancing their careers, don't forget to highlight their successes as a way to aid in recruitment and retention efforts. Highlight and celebrate a staff member's successes by placing a photo of yourself and the nurse in the local community newspaper detailing his or her professional career advancement path, and include comments about how the hospital supports the nurse.

Proven Pearls

We developed an education channel, which is a TV monitor set up in each nursing department, and we play a PowerPoint in a continuous loop, filled with various education announcements and small bits of training. But mixed in with that we have slides of our nurses' pictures and a list of excellent achievements recognizing nurses for doing well on quality improvement scores. For example, their medication verification percentages are presented next to their names. If someone achieved a new certification or finished his or her BSN or master's, it would be recognized.

—**Carolee Hager, RNC, staff education coordinator at Pratt Regional Medical Center in Pratt, KS**

Certify nursing excellence

Support professional development by encouraging the nursing staff to pursue certification in their clinical area of specialty. This support can come in many ways: paying for the certification, providing a review course of the exam on-site and free of charge, or even paying a differential on the employee's base pay to reward his or her accomplishments. It is also important for the unit and the organization to recognize the employee's successful completion of a certification program. The recognition can be:

- A banner on the employee's unit

- A mention of the employee's accomplishment in the hospital's employee newsletter

- A small party with cookies and punch

Proven Pearls

We recognize nurses who achieve certification with a dinner hosted by the nursing education and professional development shared governance council. The council has hosted this event for the past two years. It has been well received and appreciated. The catered dinner is held at the hospital and any current certified nurses are invited. The event has helped the organization keep track of nurses who have achieved certification; because nurses want to be invited they are sure to forward their certified information.

—**Debbi Sorrels, RN, MSN, Magnet Recognition Program®
project coordinator at Baptist Hospital East in Louisville, KY**

We recognize staff [members] who have gained specialty certification in our nursing newsletter.

—**Marian A. White, RN, MSN, BC, Magnet Recognition Program®
project coordinator at Memorial Hospital in Belleville, IL**

Reach the top

A strong clinical ladder or career advancement program is a great way for nurses to advance their careers but stay at the bedside.

Nursing clinical ladder programs are a way to recognize and reward staff nurses as they develop in their professional nursing practice, and they are a great way to retain nurses at the bedside by promoting professional growth through career advancement opportunities. Staff nurses see the clinical ladder program as an opportunity to advance their career goals and personal development without leaving the bedside, and as an opportunity to share their expertise at the unit and organizational levels.

RETENTION GEM: CASE STUDY

Levels on the Professional Ladder

Before Presbyterian Hospital of Dallas started offering a new clinical ladder program, it had to figure out how to handle some of the technicalities involved with offering a paid incentive program for professional development. Some of the details it had to take into consideration before implementation included:

- Payroll: Find out whether compensation bonuses could be issued in a separate check if they were not related to hourly rate pay

- Tracking mechanisms: Plan how the compensation bonuses would be coded and how to track what had been spent on advancement levels and on the program

- Transfer procedures: Plan how moving from different units and specialty areas would affect a nurse's career advancement level

The professional development program Presbyterian chose follows a traditional clinical ladder model. Levels I and II are applicable for all nurses, and Levels III and IV are for RNs who meet established criteria.

RETENTION GEM: CASE STUDY

The following are Presbyterian's four clinical ladder levels and the competency level of nurses in that category:

- Level I: entry-level nurses who depend on rules, guidelines, and supervision

- Level II: RNs who have skills in analytical thinking, problem-solving, priority-setting, and efficiency

- Level III: advanced levels of clinical nursing practice who use evidence-based practice (EBP) and advanced clinical expertise, and who teach/mentor peers

- Level IV: leaders in the clinical setting, who demonstrate outstanding performance with a commitment to EBP, fulfill unit and organizational goals, and perform high-quality care

The five-step ladder

The clinical ladder program at Franklin Square Hospital in Baltimore has five steps for career advancement: Steps 1 and 2 are for entry-level nurses, and steps 3, 4, and 5 require staff nurses to present an annual portfolio of their development. The portfolio consists of evidence such as community involvement, membership in a council, and involvement in an EBP project.

Step 4 requires nurses to obtain either a specialty certification or a BSN, and step 5 requires specialty certification and a BSN, says Kathleen Sabatier, MS, RN, Magnet Recognition Program® coordinator. Staff nurses are compensated as they move up the clinical ladder with an increase in their base salary: Step 3 brings a $1.50/hour increase, step 4 brings a $2.50/hour increase, and step five means a $3.50/hour increase.

Nurses who want to progress in the clinical ladder program can apply online, and are then mailed the application materials and a binder for collecting and presenting evidence. The credentials review task force at Franklin Square Hospital, part of the professional nursing development council, assigns a "ladder buddy" to nurses applying for steps 3 through 5 of the clinical ladder program. This buddy provides coaching throughout the portfolio development process.

Source: HCPro's Advisor to the ANCC Magnet Recognition Program®, 2007. Adapted with permission.

Proven Pearls

We are a shared governance facility and involvement is an expectation. We have a clinical ladder program and nurses are encouraged to advance up the ladder. Currently more than 50% of the nursing staff has advanced to a higher level in the clinical ladder program. Participation is discussed in the interview process with new employees, as well as the philosophy that change is good.

—Patricia Crabtree, RN, BSN, MHA, CNA, nurse manager at Saint Joseph Hospital in Atlanta

On-Site Educational Forums

Offering continuing education forums on-site and free of charge to nurses will help boost your professional staff's career development. Prepare for educational forums by selecting knowledgeable speakers (in-house or local), solid topics, refreshments, and logistics for the day. Here are a few on-site education forum ideas that you may want to try:

- Bring a qualified candidate on-site to teach nursing research and EBP to staff nurses

- Invite nurses to attend leadership programs on such topics as coaching, counseling, and managing change

- Provide programs for nurses on delegation, negotiation, and conflict management

- Demonstrate a commitment to cultural competence by providing educational programs that deal with cultural diversity in healthcare

Eat and learn

Although educational fairs can be held in monthly staff meetings, you can also open them to the entire hospital during a time many can attend—lunch!

Every few months schedule a roundtable discussion during lunch and encourage each staff member to say to the group, "These are the talents, knowledge, skills, and experience I bring to the team. This is an area in which I would like to improve my performance this next quarter. I need support/help/mentoring so I can improve. How can I get this from my peers?"

Proven Pearls

We have a lunch-n-learn. Every month a topic is picked, like documentation, peer review, or risk management, and it's open to the entire hospital. I cook the lunch and a speaker comes in for free, and it's free education for our staff.

—**Beth Kessler, RN, director on the med-surg unit at Lehigh Valley Hospital and Health Network in Allentown, PA**

The Worlds of Speaking and Publishing

As healthcare organizations are under mounting pressure to increase quality improvement, patient satisfaction, and positive outcomes, nursing conferences are looking for knowledgeable speakers to speak on pressing healthcare concerns, and publications are seeking writers to address these same issues.

Spread the news

Get the nursing staff to participate in speaking engagements about their clinical practice as a way to advance their speaking skills, share their expertise, and recognize their professional skills. Staff nurses are often very reluctant to participate in public-speaking opportunities, as they often don't have a lot of experience. One way to help nurses become accustomed to public speaking is to start them off by conducting an inservice to the unit staff.

 Nurse Retention Toolkit

If a nurse is resistant to speaking, try having him or her conduct a poster presentation at a local conference. This still serves as a great way to get the presenter in front of a new audience, and it's perhaps less intimidating than making a podium presentation to a large group.

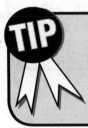

Kick it up a notch and have nurses present at a national conference. This may sound like a very large goal, but many conference-planning committees are on the lookout for new talent and new topics that have not yet saturated the speaking circuit.

Proven Pearls

As part of their goals for the oncoming year, our RNs take on small projects that reflect their positive skills. For example, I have a charge nurse who has excellent delegation skills. I asked her to present to the staff ideas on how to delegate and show respect.

—**Donna Noe, clinical manager of 2 East at Huron Valley Sinai Hospital in Commerce Township, MI**

Fame comes with the job

Provide nurses the opportunity to show off their expertise by encouraging them to publish articles in a nursing journal or newsletter. Nursing publications are constantly looking for articles with answers to complex clinical issues along with creative ways to recruit and retain staff members. So, what is your nursing unit doing that is noteworthy and "out of the box" that other nurses would like to read about?

Many publications have guidelines for submitting articles/abstracts that must be followed and can sometimes prove intimidating for the novice writer. Thus, pair the nurse with someone from within the organization who has published before and understands the process and expectations.

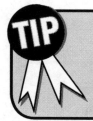

Have your department of education offer classes to nurses who would like to learn how to write articles to be published. Once staff members hear how their peers achieved a byline on an article, it becomes an attainable goal for them as well.

Most organizations also have numerous research projects taking place that staff nurses can participate in, or that prompt them to think of their own proposals for a research project, collaborate with someone who is involved formally in nursing research, or speak with someone from the organization's institutional review board to gain ideas for involvement. A lot of times the outcomes of research projects provide a good opportunity for professional advancement, and sometimes the research can be published as a scholarly article in nursing research publications.

Performance Reviews Measure Professional Development

Performance reviews must be key parts of any professional development program as they provide a forum for feedback, review, setting goals, and honest communication. No retention program can be successful without effective performance reviews, which are vital retention tools that should be part of your ongoing retention efforts to keep nurses committed to you and the organization.

An effective retention program needs performance reviews that accomplish something and that both management and the staff can trust. Before you begin a program or revitalize your existing one, consider that an effective program should clearly identify employees' strengths and weaknesses and guide them in goal-setting.

Follow these three steps when reviewing how you currently work with staff members at the time of their annual review or evaluation.

Step 1: Prepare the employee

- Send a letter or e-mail that confirms the date and time of the review

- Outline any material the employee is required to bring with him or her

- Ask the employee to review a copy of his or her job description and plan to discuss it

- Have the employee present a list of the continuing education activities in which he or she has participated during the past year

- Encourage the employee to bring copies of letters from coworkers or patients that recognize the employee's efforts as a way to demonstrate the importance of his or her role to the department and the organization

- Give the employee a worksheet to help guide him or her in setting goals (see Figure 8.1)

By working together to set goals, you set out on a communication path to try to find what inspires and motivates the nurse. When nurses know their manager supports their goals and they are asked to be a part of the solution for challenges in the department, they become team players. This feeling leads to commitment, which is your retention motivator.

Figure 8.1	**Goals Worksheet**

Name: _____

Job title: _____ Today's date: _____

Short-term goals

Professional: _____

_____

In the next year, I would like to do the following:

Add _____ to my job description.

Take _____ continuing education classes.

Work on projects related to improving _____

Long-term goals

In the next three to five years, I would like to do the following:

Have completed _____

Make these changes in my job _____

Have accomplished _____

Obtain certification in _____

Source: Shelly Cohen, RN, BS, CEN, Health Resources Unlimited, www.hru.net.. Adapted with permission.

Step 2: Prepare yourself

- Have documentation to support your discussion of both positive and negative comments. Include copies of letters or notes from the employee's peer group, evidence of time sheets with tardy dates if attendance is an issue, or incident reports from multiple occurrences of similar events.

- Have a clear perspective on what you want to communicate about the employee's work performance.

- Identify how you see the employee getting more involved in patient outcomes.

- Set a plan that includes clear expectations and timelines for changes in unacceptable behavior.

Step 3: Prepare key questions to prompt communication

- If you had the power to change just one thing about this department, what would it be?

- Is there anything you have accomplished over the past year of which I am not aware that you would like to share?

- You are a huge asset to this department, and I appreciate all of your efforts and would like to know, what motivates you to come to work every day?

- Where do you see your department heading in light of the recent issues and challenges we discussed at our last staff meeting?

- What can I, or our facility, do to help you do your job more effectively?

Proven Pearls

On my unit, I like to keep an ongoing job performance log for each employee. I try to make notes in it throughout the year documenting all the good things I see [the] staff doing. For example, whenever they volunteer to work an extra shift, read a journal article, do extra cleaning, join a committee, or just brighten someone's day, I will typically send an e-mail thanking them and then also note it on their job performance log. When it comes time for their annual performance review, I get to list all the things they have done throughout the year. Many of them tell me, "Oh, I had forgotten all about that" or "I didn't think anyone noticed," but they are pleased to know that someone noted their hard work and that it was recorded on their permanent record.

—**Debbie Smith, RNC, charge nurse, nursery/NICU at The Medical Center
at Bowling Green in Bowling Green, KY**

Reference

Cohen, S. and Sherrod, D. (2005). *A Practical Guide to Recruitment and Retention: Skills for Nurse Managers*. Marblehead, MA: HCPro, Inc.

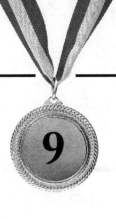

Professional Nursing Culture: Retention Benefits of Achieving Nursing's Highest Honor

LEARNING OBJECTIVES

After reading this chapter, the participant will be able to:

- Explain how the ANCC Magnet Recognition Program® relates to retention

- Identify the benefits to achieving designation

- Recognize how each of the 14 Forces of Magnetism helps retain nurses

How Designation Helps Organizations Stand Out

Did you ever think we would see the day when healthcare became this competitive? Consumers are becoming increasingly savvy regarding their care management and now realize they have numerous choices about their healthcare providers. Gone are the days when insurance plans dictated the physician you visit and the hospital you go to. Physicians and hospitals alike are striving to get the edge on the marketplace and gain loyal patients.

Everyone is working to be the provider of choice. *Quality*, *transparency*, and *state of the art* are terms we frequently hear to describe the current state of healthcare. But how can consumers know which healthcare organizations are the best? How do they know when they are admitted to the hospital that they will get the best care, as well as the best caregivers? Increasingly, more and more healthcare organizations are looking to American Nurses Credentialing Center (ANCC) Magnet Recognition Program® (MRP) designation as their mark of quality to the community. The MRP program, with its easily recognized logo and brand, is something that sends a clear message to healthcare consumers—and crucially, to employees as well. MRP designation means that the top healthcare talent works at the organization and that if you are a patient, you will get the best care possible.

Nurses and designation

The benefits of achieving MRP designation are many, but one of the keys is the attraction and retention of professional nurses. The current nursing shortage is sometimes nicknamed the "perfect storm" due to all the factors that have aligned to make this the worst shortage the United States has experienced so far. The average age of the RN is rising and there are not enough new nurse graduates to fill these positions when they retire. Schools of nursing are turning away qualified applicants because of faculty shortages, insufficient clinical sites, classrooms, and preceptors, and budget constraints.

The need to attract and retain top talent at the bedside is becoming more important than ever. Because sufficient numbers of professional nurses are essential if patients are to receive quality care, healthcare providers must seek to solve their own shortage by attracting and retaining experienced nurses.

But MRP designation is not only a useful recruitment and retention tool. High-quality nursing care makes an organization a desirable place for many other healthcare professionals, and designation can be an excellent recruitment tool for other disciplines.

The history behind the program

The ANCC developed the Magnet Recognition Program® to recognize preeminent healthcare organizations that have a high standard of nursing excellence. The MRP was started in 1983 when The American Academy of Nursing's (AAN) Task Force on Nursing Practice in Hospitals conducted a study with more than 100 hospitals to identify variables that contributed to nurse recruitment and retention. The characteristics that seemed to set those organizations apart from others, and that made them "magnets" for nurses, later became known as the 14 Forces of Magnetism.

In 1990, the proposal for the Magnet Recognition Program® was approved by the ANA Board of Directors and was expected to build upon the previous study that was conducted by the AAN. In 2002, the name of the program was officially changed to the Magnet Recognition Program®. MRP designation is the highest level of recognition the ANCC awards to organized nursing services in the national and international healthcare communities. The program recognizes healthcare organizations that demonstrate excellence in nursing practice and adherence to national standards for the organization and delivery of nursing services. Recognizing quality patient care and innovative professional nursing practice, the program provides consumers with the ultimate benchmark to measure the quality of care they can expect to receive. And it provides an avenue for nurses to practice at an organization that is dedicated to nurses.

Retain Nurses by Force

In 2008, the ANCC reorganized the 14 Forces under a new model of MRP designation. The 14 Forces are organized under five components, but the Forces still play a major role in why nurses remain at the bedside in designated organizations.

Component 1: Transformational leadership

Force 1: Quality of nursing leadership. Nurse managers take on a stronger leadership role to keep nurses happy by focusing on strategic initiatives, unit growth as a team, achievement of quality benchmarks, relationships with bedside nurses, and retention strategies.

Force 3: Management style. Nursing administrators incorporate feedback from staff members at all levels to help with communication and relationship building. This feedback is conducted through face-to-face forums, peer evaluations, and staff nurse presentations at director/manager meetings.

Component 2: Structural empowerment

Force 2: Organizational structure. MRP hospitals normally have flat organizational structures, allowing bedside nurses to be involved in decision-making, as evidenced by participation in quality, education, leadership, research, practice, recruitment, and retention councils.

Force 4: Personnel policies and programs. Personnel policies and programs are created with staff involvement. The topics of discussion include retention incentives, flexible scheduling options, mentorship programs, and certification and educational advancement.

Force 10: Community and the healthcare organization. Community presence is established through ongoing, long-term outreach programs that show the hospital's dedication to the community. This involves staff members in state nursing associations, and community events such as AIDS coalitions, a cancer society, the March of Dimes, and a multiple sclerosis society.

Force 12: Image of nursing. Staff nurses are seen as advocates to the hospital and

© 2008 HCPro, Inc.

essential to providing patient care. This is shown through nurse involvement on hospital committees, display of awards won, recognition during meetings and external events, and respect from physicians.

Force 14: Professional development. Designated hospitals seek to increase the number of certified nurses by reimbursing certification costs, improve education through tuition reimbursement and bringing courses on-site, and recognize professional advancement through a clinical ladder program where nurses can receive monetary rewards.

Component 3: Exemplary professional practice

Force 5: Professional models of care. Hospitals implement an organizationwide model of care that reflects their vision and mission. From there, units implement their care-delivery model that exemplifies the organizational model of care. Care-delivery models give nurses the responsibility and authority for the provision of direct patient care, and nurses are accountable for their own practice as well as for the coordination of care.

Force 8: Consultation and resources. Staff nurses receive peer support from within and outside the nursing division, such as nursing consultation from APNs. Other resources include staff nurses and nursing faculty collaboration on research projects, nurses as members of the hospital's ethics committee, and availability of computers or a library to support nursing research.

Force 9: Autonomy. Designated hospitals have shared governance, enabling nurses to have a voice. Staff nurses make unit-based decisions concerning clinical care, the nurse practice council is staff-driven, and nurse managers may encourage staff members to challenge care regimes that they are concerned about with the understanding that they will be supported in their decisions.

Force 11: Nurses as teachers. MRP hospitals believe that nursing knowledge is gained through experience, and it encourages its nurses to serve as teachers, both at the bedside and beyond. For example, staff nurses are preceptors to new staff members, teach survival skills to diabetics at the bedside, and mentor peers or nursing students at local colleges.

Force 13: Interdisciplinary relationships. Collaborative practice enables nurses to provide excellent care and gain a mutual respect among all disciplines. Nurses and physicians have open communication through roundtables or lunch-and-learns, and they are involved in interdisciplinary councils and research projects.

Component 4: New knowledge, innovation, and improvements

Force 7: Quality improvement. Staff nurses participate in quality improvement activities to enhance the quality of care delivered in the organization. Unit-based quality projects are staff-driven, and nurses play an active role on the nurse quality council to implement change.

Component 5: Empirical quality results

Force 6: Quality of care. Providing quality care is an organizationwide priority, and nurses perceive that they provide high-quality patient care. MRP hospitals are constantly conducting nursing research and performing evidence-based practice projects to deliver the best care; staff nurses have input into quality measures and the hospital quality initiative; and patient, nurse, and employee satisfaction survey results are benchmarked on an ongoing basis to continually look for ways to improve scores.

Benefits of Designation

MRP status is one of the highest achievements a hospital can attain in the nursing world and it recognizes the caliber of the nursing staff and the outcomes they are able to achieve. MRP designation demonstrates to nurses that the hospital recognizes the superior work they do, and it helps to build organizational commitment and loyalty. The nurses feel like key contributors to the hospital's success; most importantly, designation is an important recognition of nurses' worth to the organization.

Attaining MRP designation is beneficial to organizations in many ways, and research has identified the following nursing characteristics that are present in MRP hospitals:

- Flatter organizational structure

- Higher nurse-to-patient ratios

- Limited use of external agency personnel

- Enhanced clinical practice through research

- Flexible patient care delivery systems

- Higher percentage of BSN prepared nurses

- Investment in education for professional development

- Decreased vacancy and nurse turnover rates

- Ability to attract high-quality physicians

- Positive, collaborative, engaging work environment for all employees

Research has also shown that nurses achieve the following benefits from designation:

- Autonomy in clinical practice decision-making

- Participation in nursing leadership and organizational decision-making

- Higher RN job satisfaction

- Enhanced nurse–physician collaboration

And finally, patients see many benefits:

- Decreased length of stay

- Increased patient/family satisfaction

- Reduced family complaints

- High quality of nursing care

Attain a competitive edge

Designation means a competitive advantage in the marketplace. Research has shown that the public has more confidence in the quality of care received in a designated facility versus one that has not met the rigorous criteria to achieve the award. This can mean improved patient volumes and increased revenue. Therefore, designation is frequently used in marketing promotional campaigns to send a strong message to the public (e.g., "This facility has the best staff to provide the best patient outcomes!").

Improve patient outcomes

Achieving MRP status is known to improve patient outcomes. The program encourages continual performance assessment and improvement processes so the organization can consistently provide the highest quality of care to patients. This translates to a quicker recovery time for patients, and care that centers on their needs (patient-focused care). Research has shown that patients in designated hospitals experience a shorter length of stay, lower ICU utilization, lower mortality rates, and increased patient satisfaction.

Proven Pearls

Since Medical Center of Central Georgia in Atlanta began its MRP journey in 2002, we have seen the following positive changes:

- Decrease in vacancy rate from 25% to 8%.
- Decrease in RN turnover from around 18%–20% to about 10%–13%.
- Increase in patient satisfaction scores from 91% to 94%.
- Increase in research projects from three per year to 10–15 per year.
- Improvements in quality at the unit level, based on evidence-based practice and research, which is nurse-initiated and nurse-driven. For example:
  - Reduced hospital-acquired pressure ulcer rate by 29%
  - Reduced cardiovascular ICU blood culture contamination rate from 4.5% to 2%
  - Increased breastfeeding from 30% to 80% in neonatal population

**—Meryl Montgomery, MRP coordinator and director of learning
at Medical Center of Central Georgia in Atlanta**

It has been an impressive 10-year MRP journey with an intensive focus during the past three years. The change in our organization has been positive. Unit councils know their nursing-sensitive indicators and have created performance improvement teams to [decrease] falls, pressure ulcers, infection rates, and so on. We have offered classes for certification and our nurses are taking the initiative to attain their certification, and we plan celebrations with our CEO attending. The work with the other disciplines has initiated conversations that we have never had, such as how we can improve what we are doing to impact our patient outcomes. Our medical staff has addressed long-standing behavioral issues, and nurses and physicians consistently interact in a respectful manner. Nursing peer review reports are reviewed and acted upon with house-wide initiatives; we have the largest number of clinical ladder nurses that we have had for years; and our pressure ulcer rate is the lowest it has been in three years.

**—Cindy Kamikawa, RN, MS, CAN, vice president of nursing
and CNO at Queens Medical Center in Honolulu**

Is your organization ready?

Is your organization ready to pursue MRP designation? Help your organization assess its readiness for designation by answering the following nine questions:

1. Is the nursing organizational structure generally flat, with staff nurses involved in unit-based decision-making?

2. Do staff nurses actively participate in decision-making committees?

3. Does evidence-based practice guide nursing policies/procedures and clinical decision-making?

4. Is there an active nursing research council in place?

5. Does the organization provide opportunities for the professional growth and development of staff nurses?

6. Does the organization collect data at the unit level on nursing sensitive indicators (e.g., nurse satisfaction, falls, pressure ulcers, patient satisfaction, skill-mix, etc.)?

7. Are there committees at the nursing level (e.g., nursing practice council, nursing education council) composed of staff nurses where practice decisions are made?

8. Are there mechanisms in place to support RNs in obtaining professional certification?

9. Do the majority of staff nurses feel they have adequate staff to provide quality patient care?

Proven Pearls

At Virginia Commonwealth University Health System (VCUHS) in Richmond, VA—an American Nurses Credentialing Center Magnet Recognition Program (MRP) recipient in 2006—MRP champions wanted to educate the organization about how staff nurses exemplify the 14 Forces of Magnetism. A 10-minute video that could be shown throughout the organization was the answer.

The champions found an internal videographer who understood VCUHS's MRP culture and visited nursing units to film and interview staff nurses.

Copies of the video are available on all nursing units for review, and the video is also given to local recruiters who are speaking with student nurses interested in coming to work for the organization.

—**Rebecca Shermer, RNC, MS, clinical nurse IV, labor and delivery, and MRP champion**

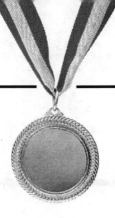

Nursing Education Instructional Guide

Target Audience

- Nurse managers

- Director/VP of Nursing and CNO

- Chief nurse executive

- Clinical Services

- Educational Services

- Administrative

- Patient Care Director/VP

- Library

- Administrator

- RNs

- Staff Development/Education

- Directors of education

Statement of need

This book helps nurse managers engage and retain bedside nurses. From low-cost and free retention tips to long-range issues that focus on career development and building a positive work environment, this book gives managers practical strategies they can use to raise their retention rates and keep their nurses engaged, committed, and loyal every day. (This activity is intended for individual use only.)

Educational objectives

Upon completion of this activity, participants should be able to:

- Identify budget-friendly ways to reward staff nurses

- Demonstrate how to build relationships with other organizational departments

- Identify Web sites that offer personalized gifts

- Recognize ways to celebrate Nurses Week

- Identify simple and free ways to reward staff

- Identify local resources to recognize staff

- Recognize ways to have fun while working

- Identify retention tips for four generations

- Identify how nurses of all generations want to be recognized

- List simple ways to recognize new nurse graduates

- Discuss strategies that help prevent new nurses from leaving

- Explain ways to provide positive feedback to new nurses.

- Identify the benefits of mentoring programs for new graduates

- Recognize ways to improve leadership skills

- Discuss how to build relationships with the staff

- Describe how to use good listening skills

- Support a relationship-building environment

- Use nursing retreats as a way to build morale and have fun

- Identify how to improve communication between nurses

- Identify steps to creating a budget

- Assess how to get buy-in for the budget from upper management

- Identify how to prepare for recruitment

- Identify ways to help nurses advance in their careers

- List ways to conduct on-site educational forums

- Explain best practices for using performance reviews as a way to retain staff members

- Explain what ANCC Magnet Recognition Program® designation is

- Identify the benefits for achieving designation

- Recognize how each of the 14 Forces of Magnetism helps retain nurses

Faculty

Bonnie Clair, BSN, RN, works as Retention Project Manager (formerly a Nurse Retention Coordinator) at CoxHealth in Springfield, MO. Lydia Ostermeier MSN, RN, CHCR, is Director of Nurse Recruitment, Retention, Workforce Development, Resource Allocation, and Customer Service at Clarian Health in Indianapolis, IN.

Nursing Contact Hours

HCPro is accredited as a provider of continuing nursing education by the American Nurses Credentialing Center Commission on Accreditation.

This educational activity for 3 nursing contact hours is provided by HCPro, Inc.

Disclosure statements

Bonnie Clair and Lydia Ostermeier have declared they have no relevant financial relationships to disclose related to the content of this educational activity.

Instructions

In order to be eligible to receive your nursing contact hours for this activity, you are required to do the following:

1. Read the book, *Nurse Retention Toolkit*

2. Complete the exam

3. Complete the evaluation

4. Provide your contact information on the exam and evaluation

5. Submit exam and evaluation to HCPro, Inc.

Please provide all of the information requested above and mail or fax your completed exam, program evaluation, and contact information to

Continuing Education Manager
HCPro, Inc.
200 Hoods Lane
P.O. Box 1168
Marblehead, MA 01945
Fax: 781/639-0179

NOTE:

This book and associated exam are intended for individual use only. If you would like to provide this continuing education exam to other members of your nursing staff, please contact our customer service department at 877/727-1728 to place your order. The exam fee schedule is as follows:

Exam quantity	Fee
1	$0
2–25	$15 per person
26–50	$12 per person
51–100	$8 per person
101+	$5 per person

Nursing education exam

Name: _____

Title: _____

Facility name: _____

Address: _____

Address: _____

City: _____ State: _____ ZIP: _____

Phone number: _____ Fax number: _____

E-mail: _____

Nursing license number: _____

(ANCC requires a unique identifier for each learner)

1. **A budget-friendly way to reward staff is by:**

    a. Giving them a raise.

    b. Shaking their hand.

    c. Attaching a handwritten thank you note to a basket filled with candy bars.

    d. Smiling as you walk by them.

2. **A low-cost strategy to build relationships between departments is by:**

    a. Having a cookie exchange.

    b. Waving when passing in the hall.

    c. Not gossiping.

    d. Giving leftovers from a potluck.

3. **A great Web site to find decorations for birthday or themed parties is:**

    a. *Baby.com*

    b. *Anniversary.com*

    c. *FunExpress.com*

    d. *Wedding.com*

4. **Managers can show nurses they are appreciated during Nurses Week by:**

   a. Giving staff one break during their 10-hour shift.

   b. Allowing a longer lunch break.

   c. Passing celebration duties off to them as you are too busy.

   d. Having a potluck meal for the unit where staff bring in their favorite dish to share.

5. **A simple and free strategy to recognize staff is by:**

   a. Handing out $10 coffee coupons.

   b. Beginning each staff meeting with staff recognition.

   c. Going to dinner at a five-star restaurant.

   d. Taking staff out for ice cream.

6. **A way to use local resources to recognize staff is by:**

   a. Taking an extravagant trip to an island.

   b. Creating a bookshelf to display upper management's awards.

   c. Placing a recruitment ad in the local newspaper.

   d. Providing a link from the hospital home page to the nursing Web site.

7. **Managers can foster a spirit of fun on the unit by:**

   a. Telling inappropriate jokes during staff meetings.

   b. Having a day where nurses pick a theme and can dress up.

   c. Teasing them in front of their peers.

   d. Making negative comments about patients.

8. **A retention technique for the silent generation is to:**

   a. Control their schedules.

   b. Ignore their knowledge and wisdom.

   c. Prepare them for retirement through classes.

   d. Place supplies in hard to reach areas.

© 2008 HCPro, Inc.

9. **Nurses of all generations enjoy being recognized by:**

    a. A "thank you" letter from managers, patients, and coworkers.
    b. A letter from their manager stating areas they need improvement.
    c. A decrease in pay.
    d. Working a double-shift with no additional benefits.

10. **Take the time to recognize new nurse graduates by:**

    a. Sending them home with a lot of paperwork to fill out.
    b. Being on vacation their first week on the job.
    c. Paging that they are new over the hospital intercom.
    d. Making a welcome bag full of goodies.

11. **Keep new nurse graduates from leaving the organization by:**

    a. Begging them to stay.
    b. Partnering them with a mentor or a buddy.
    c. Bribing them with free coffee.
    d. Assigning more patients to them.

12. **A way to provide positive feedback to a new nurse is by:**

    a. Holding evaluations at various stages during a new nurse's first year
    b. Waiting till they turn in their resignation letter.
    c. Telling them during their exit interview.
    d. Telling a peer and having him or her pass it on.

13. **Mentorship programs benefit new nurses because they:**

    a. Receive leadership, guidance, and emotional support.
    b. Receive gossip about other staff nurses.
    c. Offer an opportunity to complain about the job and the hospital.
    d. Hear everything they are doing wrong from the mentor.

14. A positive leadership strategy is to:

a. Keep your office door closed at all times.

b. Come in to work late.

c. Schedule to meet with a different staff person one day per week.

d. Take shorter lunch breaks.

15. Build relationships with staff by:

a. Recognizing their hard work once a year.

b. Telling HR they should do something nice for the nurses.

c. Having an open-door policy once every six months.

d. Knowing their favorite things such as candy, hobbies, etc.

16. One way to find what nurses really want and value is by asking:

a. Their spouse.

b. Their family and friends.

c. Them through a retention survey.

d. Their long-distance relatives.

17. Support a relationship-building environment by:

a. Encouraging staff to praise a peer.

b. Telling staff to only ask questions to upper management.

c. Promoting a silent environment.

d. Separating nurses by generations.

18. During a nursing retreat, build morale and have fun by:

a. Meditating.

b. Keeping quiet.

c. Playing human bingo.

d. Requiring alone time.

19. Improve communication between nurses on different units by:

   a. Pointing out another unit's patient satisfaction scores that are higher than your unit's.

   b. Encouraging nurses to bring their complaints about each other to you.

   c. Encouraging them to take their break away from work.

   d. Holding a forum of cluster units to discuss organizationwide goals.

20. The first step in creating a retention budget is:

   a. Gathering anecdotal evidence.

   b. Researching data.

   c. Making a wish list of retention activities.

   d. Ordering t-shirts for Nurses Week.

21. Obtain buy-in for the retention budget from upper management by:

   a. Putting together a strong business plan.

   b. Stating the budget is necessary or you will leave.

   c. Fighting with upper management to increase your chances.

   d. Gathering a petition list from staff.

22. A sensible strategy to include when preparing a retention budget is to:

   a. Build a budget without plans for recruitment needs.

   b. Divide half the budget for retention and half for recruitment needs.

   c. Plan for 100% retention.

   d. Forecast your potential recruitment needs.

23. Help nurses advance in their careers by:

   a. Not supporting them to pursue certification in their clinical specialty.

   b. Expecting them to learn new skills on their own.

   c. Partnering with a local college to bring courses onsite.

   d. Not paying for them to attend educational seminars.

24. Conduct onsite educational forums by:

    a. Expecting staff members to find the local sources.

    b. Bringing a qualified candidate onsite to teach nursing research and evidence-based practice.

    c. Asking friends, who don't understand nursing, to speak for free.

    d. Providing staff with text books to read on their own time.

25. Have an effective performance review with staff nurses by:

    a. Acknowledging only their weaknesses.

    b. Listening only to what you want to hear.

    c. Entering the review unprepared.

    d. Establishing measurable goals with them.

26. ANCC Magnet Recognition Program® designation is:

    a. A nursing excellence award.

    b. An award for elderly patients.

    c. A document to receive patient background information.

    d. A tool to monitor child births.

27. A benefit to achieving designation is:

    a. A larger nursing cafeteria.

    b. Nicer scrubs.

    c. Nursing retention.

    d. Coffee on all nursing units.

28. One way the culture of designation retains nurses is through:

    a. Assigned parking spaces.

    b. Nursing autonomy.

    c. Poor nurse-physician relationships.

    d. Larger offices.

Continuing education evaluation

Name: _____

Title: _____

Facility name: _____

Address: _____

Address: _____

City: _____ State: _____ ZIP: _____

Phone number: _____ Fax number: _____

E-mail: _____

Nursing license number: _____

(ANCC requires a unique identifier for each learner)

Date completed: _____

1. **This activity met the learning objectives stated:**

   Strongly Agree   Agree   Disagree   Strongly Disagree

2. **Objectives were related to the overall purpose/goal of the activity:**

   Strongly Agree   Agree   Disagree   Strongly Disagree

3. **This activity was related to my continuing education needs:**

   Strongly Agree   Agree   Disagree   Strongly Disagree

4. **The exam for the activity was an accurate test of the knowledge gained:**

   Strongly Agree   Agree   Disagree   Strongly Disagree

5. **The activity avoided commercial bias or influence:**

   Strongly Agree   Agree   Disagree   Strongly Disagree

6. **This activity met my expectations:**

    Strongly Agree   Agree   Disagree   Strongly Disagree

7. **Will this activity enhance your professional practice?**

    Yes   No

8. **The format was an appropriate method for delivery of the content for this activity:**

    Strongly Agree   Agree   Disagree   Strongly Disagree

9. **If you have any comments on this activity please note them here:**

10. **How much time did it take for you to complete this activity?**

Thank you for completing this evaluation of our continuing education activity!

Return completed form to:

HCPro, Inc. • Attention: Continuing Education Manager

200 Hoods Lane, Marblehead, MA 01945

Telephone: 877/727-1728 • Fax: 781/639-2982